P9-EGM-556
1/12

"This groundbreaking book offers an entirely new program for managing diabetes while maintaining a healthy lifestyle. With mindfulness as the core element, *Eat What You Love, Love What You Eat with Diabetes* is a comprehensive guidebook designed to create long-term, sustainable, and life-enhancing strategies for those who are living with diabetes. Authors Michelle May and Megrette Fletcher seamlessly integrate mindful eating concepts with cutting-edge research, anecdotal stories, visual diagrams, self-care practices, and more. The result? A comprehensive, compelling, and well-structured program that inspires, motivates, and teaches. This is a very beneficial program that is sure to increase mindful self-awareness, fulfillment, and the power of healthy choice."

> —Donald Altman, MA, LPC, author of *One-Minute Mindfulness* and *Meal By Meal*

"What Michelle May and Megrette Fletcher have done so well is to extend the benefits of mindfulness to those whose lives depend on cultivating awareness of their bodies and their actions."

> —Brian M. Shelley MD, wellness director at First Choice Community Healthcare in Albuquerque, NM

"*Eat What You Love, Love What You Eat with Diabetes* is a book that will be beneficial to anyone with a diagnosis of diabetes or insulin resistance (prediabetes). Often, a diagnosis of one of these conditions comes with dietary rules that set many into a restrictive mindset that not only takes all the joy away from eating, but could actually send them into a restrict-binge cycle with carbohydrates. This book presents a rational program to manage diabetes without anxiety. One can truly make peace with food, eating, weight, and activity."

> —Reba Sloan, MPH, LRD, FAED, licensed registered dietitian in Nashville, TN

"If you're committed to changing your relationship with food and losing weight and nothing you've tried before has stuck, look here. Michelle May and Megrette Fletcher take you on a guided tour of mindful eating. You'll begin to taste your food again and enjoy it more while being satisfied with less."

> —Riva Greenberg, author of *50 Diabetes Myths That Can Ruin Your Life* and *The ABCs Of Loving Yourself With Diabetes*

"Michelle May and Megrette Fletcher have produced a brilliantly clear resource for stopping the downward spiral into prediabetic and diabetic behavior. What a truly compassionate, humanistic, mindfulness-powered manual for fearlessly instinctive eating!"

—Pavel Somov, PhD, author of *Eating the Moment* and *Reinventing the Meal*

"Through simple but powerful psychological techniques, this lovely book demonstrates how it is possible to gain a more positive perspective on diabetes and take action towards living a healthier life. I enthusiastically recommend this book!"

—William H. Polonsky, PhD, CDE, CEO of Behavioral Diabetes Institute and associate clinical professor at the University of California, San Diego

"*Eat What You Love, Love What You Eat with Diabetes* is a revolutionary approach to eating for people working with the challenges of diabetes. This book helps transform those challenges into adventures of exploration and discovery. Too often, diabetes treatment makes people feel overwhelmed and locked in by rigid dietary restrictions. When eating is persistently flavored with anxiety, people lose track of the natural pleasure and joy of eating. This very readable book has many helpful hints and exercises to help guide people with diabetes back to a sense of balance and ease with food and eating. I enthusiastically endorse it for anyone, but especially for those with diabetes and their friends and families."

—Jan Bays, MD, pediatrician and author of *Mindful Eating*

"This dynamic duo of physician and dietitian are truly empowering readers with mindful eating principles by approaching food/eating and diabetes with awareness, not anxiety; curiosity, not criticism; and trust, not doubt. For the growing number of people with diabetes, this book offers a flexible approach to eating that is both enjoyable and sustainable by introducing nutrition with a non-restrictive, all-foods-fit perspective that works—even when you have diabetes."

—Elaine Magee, MPH, RD, author of *Tell Me What to Eat if I Have Diabetes*

"There are no food police in this skillful extension of Michelle May's book *Eat What You Love, Love What You Eat* for individuals living with diabetes. Mindful eating provides a new path to truly enjoying eating and food without struggle or guilt. The book provides the foundation for eating mindfully woven together with Megrette Fletcher's wisdom as a dietitian."

> —Jean Kristeller, PhD, developer of Mindfulness-Based Eating Awareness Training and cofounder of The Center for Mindful Eating

"These authors present a compassionate, healing approach for all those who manage diabetes on a daily basis. This easy-to-read book teaches practical, life-changing strategies for taking charge of your health and taking care of yourself in a mindful way."

> —Susan Albers, PsyD, clinical psychologist at the Cleveland Clinic and author of *Eating Mindfully* and *50 Ways to Soothe Yourself Without Food*

"*Eat What You Love, Love What You Eat with Diabetes* is a refreshing and compassionate approach to managing diabetes that uses mindfulness to empower the patient. Readers will enjoy the friendly and straightforward writing style, which offers practical tips that might be surprising."

> —Evelyn Tribole, MS, RD, coauthor of Intuitive Eating

EAT WHAT YOU LOVE
LOVE WHAT YOU EAT
WITH
DIABETES

a mindful eating program for thriving with prediabetes or diabetes

Michelle May, MD

with Megrette Fletcher, MEd, RD, CDE

New Harbinger Publications, Inc.

Publisher's Note

This publication is designed to provide accurate and authoritative information in regard to the subject matter covered. It is sold with the understanding that the publisher is not engaged in rendering psychological, financial, legal, or other professional services. If expert assistance or counseling is needed, the services of a competent professional should be sought.

Distributed in Canada by Raincoast Books

Copyright © 2012 by Michelle May & Megrette Fletcher
New Harbinger Publications, Inc.
5674 Shattuck Avenue
Oakland, CA 94609
www.newharbinger.com

Cover design by Amy Shoup; Text design by Michele Waters;
Acquired by Melissa Kirk; Edited by Nelda Street

All Rights Reserved

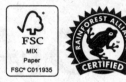

Library of Congress Cataloging-in-Publication Data

May, Michelle.
  Eat what you love, love what you eat, with diabetes : a mindful eating program for thriving with prediabetes or diabetes / Michelle May, with Megrette Fletcher.
      p. cm.
  Includes bibliographical references and index.
  ISBN 978-1-60882-245-4 (pbk. : alk. paper) -- ISBN 978-1-60882-246-1 (pdf e-book) -- ISBN 978-1-60882-247-8 (epub)
  1. Diabetes--Diet therapy. 2. Prediabetic state. I. Fletcher, Megrette. II. Title.
  RC662.M37 2012
  616.4'620654--dc23

                              2011046865

Printed in the United States of America

14   13   12

10   9   8   7   6   5   4   3   2   1

First printing

May these words unlock the prison of restrictive eating
and open the door to mindful diabetes care.

Contents

Part 4
Being Present

Part 5
Letting Go

Part 6
Acceptance

Introduction

*E*at What You Love, Love What You Eat with Diabetes might seem like a strange name for a book about type 2 diabetes. You may even be thinking, *Eating what I love is what got me into this mess in the first place!* or *I already love to eat—that's my problem!*

The truth is, although many people say they love to eat, they don't act like it. They eat too fast to even notice the taste after the first few bites, or they eat while doing other things, like watching TV, working, or driving. They eat out of habit: because it's time to; because the food looks good; or because they're stressed, bored, or any of a thousand other reasons. They may choose food they like, but their feelings of being stuffed and miserable afterward ruin the meal. These habits have serious consequences when you have prediabetes or diabetes.

You are not alone. About 25.8 million people have diabetes and 79 million people have diabetes in the United States in 2011(CDC 2011). Fifty-eight percent of people with prediabetes can prevent the onset of diabetes by making consistent lifestyle changes (NDIC 2008). As powerful as this fact is, few people can follow a restrictive diet long term. Being diagnosed with prediabetes or diabetes doesn't suddenly change that.

Why Mindful Eating?

Mindful eating is an ancient yet innovative approach to making changes. This definition of mindful eating from The Center for Mindful Eating (at www .tcme.org, cofounded by Megrette) highlights the benefits of this approach:

Mindfulness helps focus our attention and awareness on the present moment, which, in turn, helps us disengage from habitual, unsatisfying, and unskillful habits and behaviors. Engaging in mindful eating practices on a regular basis can help us discover a far more satisfying relationship to food and eating than we ever imagined or experienced before. A different kind of nourishment often emerges, the kind that offers satisfaction on a very deep emotional level.

Mindfulness is awareness of what is happening right now. While that sounds pretty simple, it's not always easy. It's common to "check out" rather than notice physical sensations, thoughts, and emotions. For example, you may be distracted by television or the Internet, preoccupied with memories of the past or fantasies about the future, or unconsciously responding to triggers you learned years earlier. The tendency to ignore and even distrust what's happening right now forces you to act out of old habits and fear instead of using the most current information to make decisions. This tendency to disconnect from what you're experiencing right now affects every aspect of your life—including your health.

How This Book Helps

Eat What You Love, Love What You Eat with Diabetes is a comprehensive, mindfulness-based guide to understanding and managing prediabetes and diabetes. This practical mind-body approach shifts the conversation from rigid nutrition rules and strict exercise regimens to awareness of beliefs, thoughts, physical states, and habits for long-term lifestyle change.

With down-to-earth language and uncommon sense, *Eat What You Love, Love What You Eat with Diabetes* offers a rare prescription for managing prediabetes and diabetes: eat mindfully and joyfully *with* diabetes. We—Michelle, a family physician, and Megrette, a certified diabetes educator and dietitian—provide strategies and insights for making conscious choices toward optimal blood glucose management.

Eat What You Love, Love What You Eat with Diabetes will help you:

- Make sustainable lifestyle change the foundation of your diabetes care

- Rediscover when, what, and how much to eat, without restrictive rules

- Embrace blood glucose monitoring with an attitude of curiosity instead of fear

- Learn the basics of nutrition in clear, practical terms

- Understand why medications are an important part of diabetes care

- Discover how to make exercise a "get to" instead of a "have to"

- Become proactive at preventing the complications associated with uncontrolled diabetes

- Experience the pleasure of eating the foods you love—without guilt or bingeing

- Develop powerful patterns of thinking so you can live the balanced, vibrant life you crave

To be clear, this book won't give you a whole new set of rules to follow. Instead, we will teach you to tap into your inner "expert." You'll learn how to become more aware of your body, your thoughts, and your feelings. You'll develop the new skills and tools that are necessary for lifelong diabetes self-management and health. We call it "uncommon sense."

How Does It Work?

Eat What You Love, Love What You Eat with Diabetes is based on Michelle's book, *Eat What You Love, Love What You Eat: How to Break Your Eat-Repent-Repeat Cycle*, which time.com called one of the "Top 10 Notable New Diet Books" of 2010 (although Michelle insists that it's a "how not to diet" book). Michelle is the founder of the Am I Hungry? Mindful Eating Workshops (www.amihungry.com), a comprehensive program, presented by hundreds of licensed facilitators and available internationally, that has helped thousands of people heal from difficult relationships with food. She also founded the Am I Hungry? Facilitator Taining Program.

Eat What You Love, Love What You Eat with Diabetes is divided into six parts, each of which is based on a key mindfulness skill: "Awareness," "Curiosity," "Nonjudgment," "Being Present," "Letting Go," and "Acceptance." As you practice these mindfulness skills, you'll notice a major shift in the way you think about your eating, your physical activity, and your self-care. This shift will also positively affect your relationships, work, and other important aspects of your life.

On this foundation of mindfulness, we reconstruct the process of diabetes self-management through a series of manageable, sustainable steps that you can master one at a time. Each of the six parts is divided into four chapters:

- **Think:** Conscious decision making using the mindful eating cycle

- **Care:** Information about diabetes and how to prevent the associated complications

- **Nourish:** Nutrition from a nonrestrictive, all-foods-fit perspective

- **Live:** Physical activity that is enjoyable and can be integrated into daily life

Think. These chapters lay the groundwork for mindful eating and diabetes management by teaching you how to gain awareness of why, when, what, how, and how much you eat and where you invest your energy. As you become more fully aware of what you believe, think, feel, and do, you'll better understand how to get the results you want. You'll build a powerful foundation of important life and diabetes management skills and find fulfilling ways to nourish your body, mind, heart, and spirit.

Care. These chapters describe diabetes basics and make the connection between self-care and prevention of future problems and complications. Using the same mindfulness-based approach as we take to eating, you'll learn to notice and observe thoughts, feelings, actions, and results. You'll see that undesirable outcomes are usually the result of restrictive, unempowered thinking. These chapters cover core topics found in the American Diabetes Association's 2011 Standards of Care and the American Association of Diabetes Educators AADE7 Self-Care Behaviors, including disease prevention, necessary testing, glucose monitoring, handling hypoglycemia and hyperglycemia, problem solving, and managing medications.

Nourish. In the past, diabetes diets were sometimes rigid, confusing, or tainted with negative messages, such as "Eating carbohydrates is bad" or "Exercise to earn the right to eat." Our nutrition chapters are written from an all-foods-fit perspective so that nutrition information is used as a tool, not a weapon. Without restrictive and complicated rules, you can use nutrition information to help you self-manage your diabetes. Ultimately, each decision is yours to make and is never wrong when you eat mindfully.

Live: You'll learn how to add physical activity to your life and *life* to your physical activity. Small changes that are gradually integrated into your lifestyle are far more powerful than one huge temporary overhaul. These small, focused suggestions are very different from the "all-or-nothing" approach of the past. We'll use the "FITT" prescription to help you write a personalized exercise prescription for increased energy, health, and risk reduction. You'll learn about exercise safety, the components of fitness, how to get started, and how to keep physical activity fun and challenging for lasting benefit.

Mindful Eating and You

Eat What You Love, Love What You Eat with Diabetes will help you discover how pleasurable it is to eat mindfully, savoring every aspect of the experience. You'll *relearn* to trust your natural ability to eat just the right amount of food—and meet your other needs in more fulfilling ways. You'll learn to eat the foods you love without guilt or overeating. You'll find joy in movement and be amazed at your body's capacity to grow stronger and more flexible.

This will be a very personal journey. You'll bring your own experiences, thoughts, feelings, and beliefs to the table. Every choice you make is an opportunity to experience and better understand why you do the things you do and to choose differently next time if it will serve you better. Let us emphasize that this will be a learning process. For this approach to be effective, perfection isn't necessary. Be kind and patient with yourself; the freedom and enjoyment you'll discover are well worth it. We have both experienced the profound effect of mindfulness on the experience of eating. We are excited to share these concepts and skills with you!

PART 1

Awareness

What is necessary to change a person is to change his awareness of himself.

—Abraham Maslow

CHAPTER 1

Think:
Why Do I Eat?

Whether you have been told you're at risk for diabetes, have been recently diagnosed with diabetes, or have had diabetes for years, you may feel motivated, scared, overwhelmed, or even angry. You may wonder, *How do I live with this?—I mean* really *live with this?*

Think of your choices concerning eating, exercise, self-care, medications, and other factors affecting your diabetes as a pendulum. On one side, during the times when you're highly motivated to stay healthy, you try very hard to stay in control of everything you can. You try to make perfect food choices, even when it leaves you feeling deprived or left out. While this is admirable, it's not sustainable. When your motivation wanes (for reasons we'll explore later), you may lose control. When you feel out of control, you may make decisions despite the known consequences, such as eating too much even though you know it will wreak havoc with your blood glucose levels. This leaves you feeling guilty, ashamed, or discouraged, which compounds the problem, resulting in even worse feelings of deprivation and frustration. If you've ever dieted to lose weight or tried to make other important changes in your lifestyle, you've probably experienced these two extremes. Why? Because this pendulum swings between two extremes: in control and out of control.

Our approach to diabetes self-management isn't about being *in control*. It's about being *in charge*. Instead of seeing your pendulum swing wildly from one extreme to the other, we want to help you find balance. We'll show you how to use mindfulness to take charge of your decisions. No perfection needed.

What Is Mindfulness Anyway?

At its simplest, mindfulness is awareness of the present moment. Instead of just telling you about it, we'd like you to experience mindfulness for yourself right now. Stop reading for a moment and pay attention to your body in your seat right now. Simply notice how it feels. What are you aware of? If you notice that you're uncomfortable, what could you change to feel more comfortable? Could you shift positions? Get a drink? Grab a blanket?

You may be thinking, *Huh? That sounds too simple! All I have to do is pay attention? Besides, how can being more aware help my diabetes?* Focusing on the information available to you right now will better enable you to make self-care decisions.

Admittedly it isn't always this easy, since paying attention requires practice. The challenge is that many of us have learned to disconnect and ignore what we are experiencing right now. We live in the past (*I should have* …) or the future (*What if* …), or distract ourselves with TV, work, food—even our own thoughts! Our tendency to overlook and even distrust our present experience forces us to replay past habits and fears of the future rather than use the most current information to make decisions.

We'll build on your awareness by introducing other mindfulness skills, such as curiosity, nonjudgment, being present, letting go, and acceptance. With mindfulness, you'll notice a major shift in the way you think about physical activity, self-care, and even your relationships and other aspects of your life.

Hungry for Answers

One of the primary tools that will help you improve your awareness is the mindful eating cycle, but before we introduce it, let's look at three common eating patterns: instinctive eating, overeating, and restrictive eating.

Instinctive Eating

Think of someone who manages her eating effortlessly and seems to stay within her healthy weight range naturally. Perhaps you're thinking of your spouse, a friend, a child, or even yourself in the past. What characteristics and traits does this person have? Why does he eat? What role does food play in his life? Think of his eating patterns—what, how often, and how much does he eat? How physically active is he? Here's how Cheryl describes her husband, Roger:

Roger never worries about his weight. He weighs about the same as the day we got married. He just eats when he's hungry and stops when he's full. I mean, he loves food but doesn't seem to think about it or talk about it all the time like I do. I've seen him turn down a great dessert just because he's not hungry. Geez! He also loves to play tennis and golf. I've noticed that he's more careful about what he eats since his dad had that heart attack.

Overeating

Think of somebody who has difficulty following a healthy meal plan. It may be you or someone you know well. Mark is fairly typical of a lot of people who struggle with this.

My wife, Julie, and I have been overweight since our kids were born, but it gets worse every year. Food has become the background music to our lives. Every social event and form of entertainment has something to do with food. I eat by the clock and when I'm under stress at work. I'm one of the original members of the "clean plate" club. Look out, all-you-can-eat buffets!

Our wake-up call came last year, when I was diagnosed with type 2 diabetes. The doctor said Julie's blood sugar was borderline high, too, and that it was just a matter of time before she developed diabetes if she didn't do something. We went to one diabetes class and read a bunch of stuff on the Internet, so I think I understand the whole carb thing. I just don't want to count everything I eat or give up all my favorite foods.

Restrictive Eating

Now think of someone with diabetes who tries to follow the rules perfectly. Here's how Marlise describes it:

Since I was diagnosed with type 2 diabetes earlier this year, I feel like my whole life revolves around numbers: my blood sugar, my hemoglobin A1c, my blood pressure, my cholesterol, my weight, and how many grams of carbohydrate I eat. I know I need to pay attention to these things, but it reminds me of my old diet days. That really scares me because I could never stick to one for very long. It seemed like I was always thinking about food, especially what I wasn't allowed to eat. I even hate to exercise because it feels like I'm punishing myself for eating. I worry that I won't be able to stay in control and will end up blind, on dialysis, or even dead!

The Mindful Eating Cycle

Do you recognize your eating patterns in one or more of these examples? Let's take a closer look at each one, using the mindful eating cycle as a way to understand how you make conscious or subconscious decisions about eating and how each decision affects the other choices you make.

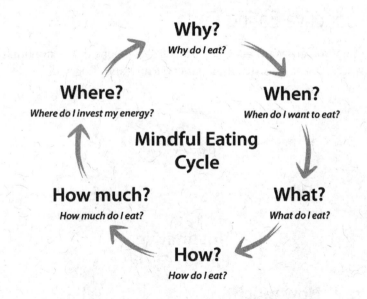

Figure 1.1

The mindful eating cycle consists of six questions to increase your awareness about your eating decisions; this cycle will help you notice why, when, what, how, and how much you eat and where you invest your energy.

Why? *Why do I eat? What drives my eating at any given time?*

When? *When do I want to eat? When do I think about eating? When do I decide to eat?*

What? *What do I eat? What do I choose from all the available options?*

How? *How do I eat? How, specifically, do I get the food I've chosen into my body?*

How much? *How much do I eat? How much fuel do I consume?*

Where? *Where do I invest my energy? That is, where does the fuel I've consumed go?*

Let's apply the mindful eating cycle to the three patterns of eating to better understand what's really going on. (To discover your own eating patterns, visit www.amihungry.com/quiz.shtml to take the eating cycle assessment.)

Instinctive Eating Cycle

Here's how you answer the six fundamental questions in the mindful eating cycle when you eat instinctively, as Cheryl's husband, Roger, did.

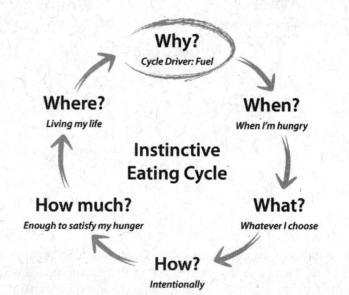

Figure 1.2

Why? Your cycle driver is fuel. Your body's need for fuel is your primary reason for eating. Hunger guides you to decide when and how much to eat.

When? When your body needs fuel, it triggers the sensations that tell you you're hungry. You decide when to eat based on how hungry you are, but you also consider other factors, like convenience, social norms, and the availability of appetizing food. Although you occasionally eat even when you're not hungry, you don't feel guilty, just full, so you don't eat again right away.

What? Your choices are affected by your preferences, awareness, and knowledge about how nutrition affects your health, as well as what foods are available. You naturally seek balance, variety, and moderation in your eating. In an instinctive eating cycle, you don't use rigid rules to decide what to eat, so you don't judge yourself for what you eat. Eating is usually pleasurable, but food doesn't hold any particular power over you.

How? You eat intentionally and with purpose. Since you're eating to satisfy hunger and nourish your body, you pay attention to the food and your body's signals.

How much? You decide how much food to eat by how hungry you are, how filling the food is, how soon you'll eat again, and other factors. When your hunger is satisfied, you usually stop eating—even if there's food left. You recognize that being too full is uncomfortable and unnecessary.

Where? Your energy goes toward living your life. You can direct your physical energy toward your activities during work, play, exercise, and even rest. You can focus your mental energy on your daily tasks and goals. You can focus your emotional and spiritual energy on your relationships and life purpose. Any leftover fuel you consume is stored until needed.

Once the fuel you've consumed is depleted or stored, the signs of hunger return, triggering your desire to eat again. The instinctive eating cycle repeats itself perhaps three or four times a day or every few hours, depending on what and how much you eat and how much fuel you need on a particular day.

Overeating Cycle

Here's how you answer the six fundamental questions in the mindful eating cycle when you are in a pattern of overeating, like Mark and Julie were.

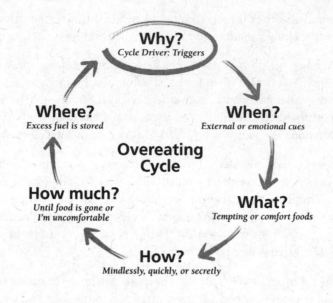

Figure 1.3

Why? Your cycle drivers are your triggers; that is, eating provides temporary distraction or pleasure. For example, if the trigger is boredom, eating distracts you and gives you something to do for a little while. If the trigger is a big tray of brownies, eating one or two might be pleasurable for a few moments. The distraction or pleasure is initially satisfying, so you eat more than you need, which drives the overeating cycle, despite the immediate effect on your blood glucose levels or the long-term effect on your health.

When? Your desire to eat is triggered by conscious or subconscious physical, environmental, and emotional triggers. Examples of physical triggers are thirst, fatigue, and pain. Environmental cues, such as time of day, appetizing food, or certain activities associated with food, may trigger your urges to eat. Emotions, such as stress, boredom, guilt, loneliness, anger, and happiness, may also trigger eating. Sometimes hunger triggers the initial urge to eat, but then environmental and emotional cues lead to overeating. If you're in the habit of eating for all these reasons, when do you feel like eating? All the time!

What? The types of food you choose to eat in response to triggers other than hunger are probably foods that are convenient, tempting, and comforting. For example, if you're at a ball game, you might eat a hot dog, a jumbo pretzel, or a plate of nachos, even though you aren't hungry and you know it will make your blood glucose levels too high. If your trigger is stress, you might choose one of your "comfort" foods, like chocolate or potato chips. You are less likely to choose nutritious foods in an overeating cycle since you're not eating in response to your body's physical needs.

How? In the overeating cycle, you may eat mindlessly, automatically, quickly, or secretly. You may eat or continue eating whether you're hungry or not. You might unconsciously grab a handful of candy or nuts from a bowl as you pass by. You might eat while you're distracted by watching TV, driving, working, or talking on the phone. You might eat secretly or quickly to finish before someone catches you. You might feel guilty about eating so that you aren't able to fully enjoy it. Eating this way is not very satisfying physically or emotionally.

How much? If hunger doesn't tell you to start eating, what tells you to stop? In an overeating cycle, the amount of food you eat depends on how much food you've been served or how much is in the package. You might eat until you feel bad or get interrupted. All too often, you feel uncomfortably full, miserable, or even numb after eating instead of content and satisfied. And your blood glucose levels show it!

Where? When you eat food your body didn't ask for, your blood glucose levels may rise out of the target range. The excess fuel you've consumed is stored in the form of body fat for later use. This extra body fat increases your insulin resistance, the hallmark of type 2 diabetes. You might feel self-conscious or less energetic and, as a result, might not feel like being physically active. Lack of physical activity decreases your metabolism, resulting in additional weight gain and potential worsening of diabetes. All of this can leave you feeling guilty and frustrated, perhaps leading to more emotional triggers and overeating.

When you ignore your true needs and eat instead, you feel disconnected and out of control. When you eat for reasons other than hunger, the distraction and pleasure are only temporary. Consequently, you have to eat more to feel better, feeding a vicious cycle.

Restrictive Eating Cycle

Here's how you answer the six fundamental questions in the mindful eating cycle when you're in a restrictive eating pattern, as Marlise was.

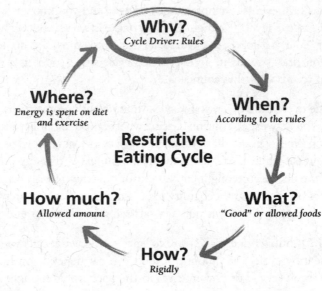

Figure 1.4

Why? Your cycle is driven by rules that determine when, what, and how much to eat to manage your blood glucose levels. When you're in a restrictive eating cycle, numbers or how well you've followed the rules determines how you feel about yourself on a particular day.

When? The rules determine whether or not you're allowed to eat: for example, *Eat every three hours* or *Never eat after 7:00 p.m.* These rules serve the purpose of externally limiting your intake. In these examples, eating by the clock stabilizes your blood glucose levels to prevent you from getting hungry, so theoretically, your eating will be easier to control. Prohibiting eating in the evening prevents eating due to triggers like boredom, watching TV, or loneliness. But these rules place artificial constraints on your eating that don't necessarily honor your body's natural hunger rhythms—and they don't address the real reasons why you want to eat in the first place.

What? You are supposed to eat only the "good" foods allowed on your meal plan. You may have to resist your favorite "sinfully delicious" foods or avoid situations and places where your forbidden foods would just tempt you. Certain foods are treated as special. These powerful foods must be substituted, calculated, earned, or eaten only on "cheat days." In the restrictive eating cycle, choosing the right food is very important, because when your choice is good, you're good. But when your choice is bad, you're bad.

How? You may believe that you need to be very structured or even rigid in your eating: weighing, measuring, counting, and writing everything down. But trying to follow rules like choosing "good" foods may cause you to feel deprived, while breaking the rules and choosing "bad" foods can cause you to feel guilty.

How much? You eat the allowed amount since the quantity of food is predetermined by rules that limit the amount of food you can have. These rules prevent you from eating too much or too little food, based on the assumption that you don't have the ability to consume an appropriate amount of food without following a set of strict rules.

Where? The restrictive eating cycle requires a great deal of mental and emotional energy. As in the instinctive eating cycle, your body will use whatever fuel it needs for work, play, exercise, and rest, but if you're eating more "healthy" foods than your body needs, the excess will still be stored. If you're significantly undereating, your body may attempt to conserve as much fuel as possible by lowering your metabolism. You may spend a lot of your energy figuring out how to get the most food while staying within the confines of your diet. Furthermore, while exercise is important for glucose management and overall health and fitness, in the restrictive eating cycle, exercise is sometimes used to earn the right to eat, to punish yourself for overeating, or to pay penance for eating a bad food.

While other people admire your willpower and self-control, many of your thoughts, feelings, and activities revolve around food, exercise, and weight. When you're dependent on rules to drive your eating cycle, you may neglect other social, emotional, and spiritual aspects of your life.

Yo-Yo Dieting with Diabetes

It's common for people to shift back and forth between overeating and restrictive eating cycles. You might switch cycles over the course of weeks or months, or you might move rapidly from one cycle to the other in the same day or even in the same meal. You start out with good intentions but quickly lose control. In weight management, this pattern is known as yo-yo dieting, but it's also very common in people with diabetes.

The problem is that a yo-yo is either up or down. You are either in control or out of control: tightly wound up in rules or unraveling toward the bottom again. There's no real in-between.

That brings us back to the pendulum. Instead of trying to stay *in control* of your eating, you will be guided to find the middle ground through mindfulness. Tapping into your awareness of your physical state, your thoughts and feelings, and the effects of your choices, you'll discover how to be *in charge* of your diabetes.

We'll show you how to use the fundamental information delivered by your hunger and fullness cues to determine when to eat, what kind of food satisfies you, and how much food you need. You don't have to eliminate your favorite foods, and you don't need an endless supply of willpower and self-control. You'll discover that it's possible to balance eating for nourishment with eating for enjoyment. Eating will become pleasurable again, free from guilt and deprivation. You'll have the tools to manage your diabetes no matter where you are or what you're doing: celebrating the holidays, doing business over lunch, or relaxing on vacation.

We'll also explore why you sometimes want to eat when you're not hungry. This awareness will give you the opportunity to meet your other needs more effectively. You'll also learn to trust your ability to make healthful decisions about physical activity and self-care, not because you have to but because you want to. Little by little, you'll discover new tools and energy for a more balanced, satisfying, and vibrant life. This is true diabetes self-management.

CHAPTER 2

Care:
Understanding Diabetes

I t can be scary to be diagnosed with a serious condition like prediabetes or diabetes. You may already know a lot about it, or perhaps it's a big black hole right now. Either way, this chapter will lay an important foundation for helping you to understand what lies ahead. The good news is that there's a lot you can do to care for yourself and stay well. The first step in taking charge is to understand diabetes.

What Is Diabetes?

Diabetes is a disorder of *metabolism*: the way the body uses digested food for growth and energy. To understand diabetes, let's first look at what happens when everything is working normally.

Just like your car, your body needs fuel to function. Your body's main form of fuel is *glucose* (sometimes referred to as "sugar"). When you eat, your body digests the food to be used for fuel and nutrients. The carbohydrates you eat are broken down to glucose, which floats in your bloodstream where it's ready to be used for energy or stored for later use. This is where the term "blood glucose" or "blood sugar" comes from. The level of glucose available in your bloodstream is closely regulated by various hormones, including insulin. *Insulin* is produced by the beta cells of the *pancreas*, an organ located behind your stomach. It may be helpful to think of insulin as a key that unlocks the cells to let glucose in.

When the level of glucose in your blood rises after you eat, insulin is released from your pancreas. Insulin moves glucose into the cells, where it can be used for energy, and stimulates your liver to make *glycogen* out of any excess glucose. Within three to four hours after you eat, your blood glucose and insulin levels return to baseline. If you don't eat (for example, while you are sleeping), the glucose stored as glycogen is released to keep your blood glucose level in the optimal range.

With diabetes, your body doesn't make enough insulin or can't use insulin properly, so glucose levels are high. In *type 1 diabetes*, the body's own immune system destroys the insulin-producing beta cells in the pancreas, causing it to stop making insulin so that there are no "keys" to let glucose into the cells. This requires for insulin to be administered immediately in order to bring glucose levels back down to a safe level. This is the least common type of diabetes.

With *type 2 diabetes*, your body resists the effects of insulin and is unable to produce enough insulin to maintain a normal glucose level. Type 2 diabetes is the most common form of diabetes, accounting for over 90 percent of all cases (CDC 2011). Although type 2 diabetes primarily affects adults, growing numbers of children have this form of diabetes.

Having diabetes puts you at risk for other problems, such as heart disease, circulation problems, and eye and kidney disease. In chapter 14, we'll talk about why these complications happen, how to watch out for them, and, most important, how to prevent them.

What Went Wrong?

While the cause is not fully understood, type 2 diabetes results from a series of problems, the first being *insulin resistance*. Just as it sounds, the fat, muscle, and liver cells resist the effects of insulin; in other words, the insulin "keys" don't fit. It's almost as if someone changed the locks and didn't tell the pancreas. The pancreas initially compensates for insulin resistance by producing more insulin—making more keys—which results in high insulin levels, or *hyperinsulinemia*. These high insulin levels promote fat storage and inhibit fat burning, causing weight gain. Eventually, the pancreas cells "burn out" and stop making enough keys (insulin) to keep up, so blood glucose levels rise. Insulin resistance may be present for five to ten years before the glucose levels are high enough to qualify for a diabetes diagnosis. By that time, the pancreas has lost about 50 percent of its ability to make insulin.

Insulin resistance is also associated with high blood pressure, abnormal levels of cholesterol and triglycerides in the blood, and obesity. Insulin resistance increases the risk of type 2 diabetes and cardiovascular disease. Cardiovascular disease is the leading cause of death in people with diabetes.

Let's see if insulin resistance is starting to make sense: When your cells need fuel, you feel tired and hungry. You eat, but the fuel (glucose) can't get into the cells easily due to insulin resistance, so it builds up in your bloodstream, causing your blood glucose level to rise. This makes you thirsty, so you drink more, which causes you to urinate more than normal (often at night). The cells still need fuel, so you still feel hungry. These three classic symptoms of diabetes—eating more, drinking more, and peeing more—are called "the polys": *polyphagia*, *polydipsia*, and *polyuria*. Unfortunately, many people do not have any symptoms at all. It is estimated that in 2011, seven million people with diabetes had not been diagnosed (CDC 2011).

Because of insulin resistance, you may be eating more and storing more fat, both of which can lead to increased insulin resistance. Having diabetes can also make you feel really tired. Think about all of the work your cells do: they keep your immune system working, help your body to repair damage, and generate energy so that you can live your life. When you have insulin resistance or diabetes, your cells are trying to do all of this work with less and less fuel. The glucose is in the bloodstream outside the cells, waiting for the body to sort through all the extra keys to find the right insulin key to unlock the few locks (channels) that allow fuel (glucose) into your cells.

Further, if you are inactive, the number of locks decreases; the fewer the locks, the fewer ways for glucose to get into the cells. Inactivity may also contribute to weight gain and increased insulin resistance. This combination of problems creates a vicious downward spiral. Fortunately, once you are aware of what's going on, and take steps to correct or deal with the underlying problems, you can change direction.

How Do You Know If You Have It?

With type 1 diabetes, the symptoms of excess hunger and thirst, increased urination, fatigue, and weight loss come on really fast. In type 2 diabetes, the blood glucose levels rise slowly. As a result, you may not realize that something is wrong right away, or you may blame the symptoms on age, weight, lifestyle, stress, or other issues.

There are a number of factors that increase your risk of developing type 2 diabetes. People with one or more of these risk factors should be screened for diabetes:

- Age over forty-five years

- Family history of type 2 diabetes (especially a first-degree relative, such as a parent or sibling)

- High-risk race or ethnicity: Latino, Native American, African American, Asian American, or Pacific Islander

- Obesity

- Sedentary or inactive lifestyle

- Low HDL (less than 35 mg/dL)

- High triglycerides (over 250 mg/dL)

- High blood pressure (greater than or equal to 140/90 mm Hg or on medication)

- Diagnosis of gestational diabetes during a pregnancy

- Giving birth to a baby weighing more than nine pounds

- Women with polycystic ovarian syndrome (PCOS)

- *Acanthosis nigricans*, a condition that causes dark, thickened skin around the neck or armpits

- A diagnosis of prediabetes (explained shortly)

A normal blood glucose level should be less than 100 milligrams per deciliter (mg/dL) when you haven't eaten for eight hours. This is called *fasting plasma glucose* (FPG). Based on "Standards of Medical Care in Diabetes—2011," by the American Diabetes Association (ADA 2011), you have diabetes if your FPG measures above 126 mg/dL. Another way to diagnose diabetes is with a blood test called *hemoglobin A1c* (HbA1c or A1C for short). An A1C tells you what your blood glucose has been, on average, over the last three months. A normal A1C is less than 5.7 percent; an A1C above 6.5 percent means you have diabetes (ibid).

People with an FPG between 101 and 126 mg/dL, or an A1C between 5.7 and 6.4, have *prediabetes* (ibid.). Having prediabetes means that you have a high risk of developing diabetes and cardiovascular disease in the future. Whether you're at risk for diabetes or have been diagnosed with prediabetes, you have an opportunity to take action—by improving your diet, increasing your activity level, and losing a modest amount of weight (7 percent of your body weight)—to prevent, or at least delay, the development of diabetes.

What Do You Do about It?

While some of the risk factors for diabetes can't be changed, the Diabetes Prevention Program (DPP) proved that by adopting consistent lifestyle changes, many people diagnosed with prediabetes were able to prevent the progression to diabetes (NDIC 2008). What you do *does* make a difference. One small step in the right direction can begin to reverse a downward spiral.

If you already have diabetes, you may wonder whether it can be cured. Diabetes is considered a chronic condition. While there is no cure, you can do a lot to improve your health and energy; keep your blood glucose, lipids, and blood pressure in the target ranges; and decrease the problems caused by diabetes. The focus shifts to managing the condition while living and enjoying your life.

How Does Mindful Eating Help?

Although there's no simple formula for managing diabetes, mindfulness can help you stop the downward spiral of overeating, inactivity, weight gain, elevated blood glucose, fatigue, and worsening insulin resistance. Becoming more mindful shifts your focus from *What do I do?* to *How do I feel?*

The serious complications from diabetes don't show up right away, so it may be challenging to stay motivated to avoid problems in the future. Your real motivation to make changes to your lifestyle, and take medication if necessary, is to feel good now. That's what Gary did:

Thinking back, I know I didn't feel good, but I could always explain it away. It amazes me that I could even function at work. I really didn't know how bad I felt until I started taking care of myself. I am so happy to finally feel good again and will do what it takes to stay this way.

Mindful eating increases your awareness of why, when, what, how, and how much you eat. By helping you see eating patterns, recognize triggers, and discover how eating affects your blood glucose, you'll begin to see food in a new way. When food is no longer the enemy, you can observe your thoughts, feelings, actions, and results without judgment, guilt, or shame. You'll replace fear, anxiety, and doubt with curiosity, trust, and pleasure. You'll learn how to nurture your body, mind, heart, and spirit. Here's how Tess described it:

> When I was counting and measuring my food, I made sure to eat every last bite, but even then, I never felt satisfied. I worried about diabetes and food all the time. This preoccupation only made things worse. When I learned to eat mindfully, I stopped worrying and could focus on eating what I needed.

We hope this book will unlock the many mysteries of diabetes and help you discover a positive and effective way to care for yourself.

CHAPTER 3

Nourish:
Masterpiece or
Paint-by-Number?

P ause for a moment to notice what you are thinking and feeling. We'll wait. You might now be aware of any number of different thoughts and feelings: boredom (*I already know this*), resistance (*I don't want to learn about carbs*), fear (*Uh-oh, they're going to tell me I can't eat sugar*), excitement (*They're finally going to tell me what to eat!*), determination (*I'm going to do it right this time*), confusion (*I thought mindful eating was just paying attention! Now I have to know stuff?*), or something else.

No matter what you noticed, accept your thoughts and feelings as they are. Then ask yourself, *Do these thoughts and feelings reflect experiences and habits that were helpful or unhelpful to me in the past?* Rather than staying stuck in old, habitual patterns, you can use awareness and curiosity, which allow you to move forward consciously and discover new ways to think about your health.

Consumed

We live in a society consumed with dieting. New fad diets scream at us from magazines and books, talk shows and news programs, commercials and testimonials, doctors' offices and health food stores. Paradoxically, obesity and diabetes are at an all-time high. Clearly, diets are not the answer.

Most health experts now agree that making sustainable lifestyle changes should be the primary goal. In 2002, the DPP (NDIC 2008) studied over three thousand participants who were overweight and diagnosed with prediabetes. They examined whether modest weight loss through dietary changes and increased physical activity or treatment with the oral diabetes drug metformin (Glucophage) could prevent or delay the onset of type 2 diabetes. Participants in the lifestyle intervention group—those receiving intensive individual counseling and motivational support on effective diet, exercise, and behavior modification—reduced their risk of developing diabetes by 58 percent. Participants taking metformin reduced their risk of developing diabetes by 31 percent. The DPP's results indicate that millions of high-risk people can delay or avoid the onset of diabetes by losing a modest amount of weight through diet and exercise. Other research shows that even a 5 percent weight loss can reduce your risk of diabetes, high blood pressure, high cholesterol, heart disease, arthritis, and some types of cancers (Cummings, Parham, and Strain 2002). In addition, an intensive lifestyle intervention can produce sustained weight loss and improvements in fitness, glycemic control, and cardiovascular disease risk factors in individuals with type 2 diabetes (The Look AHEAD Research Group 2010).

The challenge is that our diet-obsessed culture often confuses healthy lifestyle changes with restriction. As you think about the restrictive eating cycle, it's easy to see the importance of understanding the difference.

Your Picture of Health

The blurring of the line between healthy eating and restrictive dieting is the difference between a work of art and a paint-by-number. Either way, you end up with a nice picture—until you get up close to take a look.

Healthy Eating vs. Restrictive Dieting	
Healthy	Restrictive
In charge	In control
Nourishment	Diet
Fuel	Calories
Quality	Points
Healthy	Thin
Aware	Preoccupied
Conscious	Consumed
Mindful	Vigilant
Information	Dogma
Guide	Rules
All foods fit	Good foods vs. bad foods
Balance	Perfection
Variety	Temptation
Moderation	Deprivation
Choosing	Earning
Deciding	Rationalizing
Flexible	Rigid
Hunger based	By the clock
Comfort	Portion sizes
Physical activity	Penance
Introspective	Smug
Effortless	Willpower
Trust	Fear
Learning	Failing
Self-acceptance	Condemnation
Enjoyment	Guilt
Pleasure	Shame
Freedom	Bondage

Strategies: Create Your Masterpiece

Choose how you want to create *your* work of art by getting rid of *Restrictive eating is healthy* thoughts. Here are ten specific steps you can take:

1. Let go of the belief that you are incapable of managing your eating without rigid rules. Find role models, health care providers, magazines, and a support system that don't propagate that belief.

2. Filter everything you read, hear, and say about eating by asking, *Is this restrictive in nature?* You might be surprised by how pervasive restrictive messages really are.

3. Become more aware of your thoughts. It may also help to keep a journal to capture the essence of your beliefs, thoughts, feelings, and choices. When you notice restrictive messages, gently replace them with true, healthy thoughts. You'll have plenty to choose from by the time you reach the end of this book!

4. Remember, all foods can fit into a healthy diet if you allow balance, variety, and moderation to guide you.

5. Banish the words "good" and "bad" from your thoughts and speech, as in *I was good at dinner last night* or *Fast food is bad.*

6. Use nutrition information as a tool, not a weapon. It shouldn't be used to deprive yourself of certain foods, restrict yourself from ingredients like fat or carbohydrates, force you to ignore your body's signals about what it wants and needs, or make you feel guilty when you eat something you really, really want.

7. Let go of the belief that you need to eat perfectly. Just make the healthiest choices you can *without* feeling deprived.

8. Accept that sometimes you'll regret certain choices you've made; that's part of a healthy lifestyle. When you don't get caught up in guilt and shame, you're able to learn from your experiences.

9. Repeat this thought frequently: *I'm in this for the long haul. I can learn to trust and nourish myself without restriction.*

10. Apply all these ideas to your beliefs and thoughts about exercise too.

As you can see, this approach doesn't rely on willpower or, more accurately, *won't power*. As you replace restrictive and complicated diet rules with a solid foundation of nutrition information, you'll be in charge of making choices that express your individuality, preferences, and lifestyle. Create your own masterpiece!

CHAPTER 4

Live:
Change Your Mind

J ust as your thoughts about food affect your decisions about eating, your thoughts about exercise have a powerful impact on your decisions about physical activity. Although exercise is one of the most powerful tools available for improving your health and managing your blood glucose, for many people the word "exercise" conjures up negative thoughts and feelings. It's important to become aware that what you believe and think (even unconsciously) causes you to feel a certain way, which causes you to do certain things, which ultimately leads to specific results.

If you believe that fitness is important but are not very active or exercising regularly, you probably have negative and limiting beliefs that keep you from doing it. In other words, your thoughts become self-fulfilling prophecies. Since your results usually reinforce your beliefs and thoughts, this causes a self-perpetuating loop.

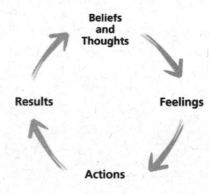

Figure 4.1

It's common for people to try to change the actions and results they don't like without first recognizing and dealing with the beliefs, thoughts, and feelings that led to those unwanted actions and results in the first place. Julie gave this example:

Whenever I saw someone who looked really fit, I thought about how long it would take me to get to that point. It seemed so unreachable that I felt totally overwhelmed and paralyzed. Needless to say, I just never seemed to get started. Then, one day, I realized my thoughts were keeping me stuck, so I changed my mind. Instead of thinking, I'll never get to that point!, *I trained myself to think,* No matter how long it will take me to get in shape, that time will pass anyway. I'll either be closer to my goals—or still right where I am right now. It's up to me. *That was the shift that got me moving.*

If you don't like your results, ask yourself what you were thinking first. Thinking thoughts that lead to undesirable results is a habit—one that you can change through awareness. Granted, it's not always easy to recognize when a thought is driving unwanted results, especially if you've been thinking a particular way for a long time. As you become aware of thoughts that lead to unwanted results, it's important to avoid judging yourself for them. Remember, it's a loop, so feeling bad or blaming yourself only leads to negative feelings.

You have the power to change the thoughts that aren't working for you. When you change your thoughts, you change your results. Next, we'll explore examples of common limiting thoughts about exercise and help you develop new, more powerful ways of thinking.

Negative vs. Positive

I know I should exercise, but I hate it, so I just can't seem to make myself do it. The negative thoughts and feelings can be heard in the words "should," "hate," and "make myself." These thoughts and feelings come from negative past experiences, like being chosen last for teams, having to do boring exercise routines, and experiencing discomfort or pain from doing too much, too fast. Some people only exercise when they are trying to lose weight, so they think of exercise as a punishment for overeating.

I enjoy becoming more physically active each day may be a good replacement thought. It helps you focus on all the great things physical activity does for you and how wonderful you feel. Find fun physical activities that suit your personality and lifestyle. Most important, start slowly and allow your body to adjust gradually and comfortably. It will be different this time if you think it will be.

Limiting vs. Encouraging

I don't know if exercise is really worth the effort is a limiting thought. Most people know that physical activity is very important, yet many people choose to lead sedentary lives—and even more find it difficult to start an exercise program or stick with it.

Thoughts like *I deserve all the amazing benefits I get from being physically active* are encouraging. Exercise has many well-documented health and psychological benefits. It lowers blood pressure and blood glucose levels, improves cholesterol and energy levels, enhances mood and sense of well-being, and helps people live longer. If you could get all that in a pill, everyone would want a prescription.

Exercise also helps you reconnect with your physical body. You may be surprised to experience great joy in movement and your ability to function optimally in your life. Exercise is not a means to an end but an end, in and of itself.

Scarcity vs. Abundance

I don't have time is a scarcity thought. Time is a real issue for many people, but the reality is that we all have exactly the same amount of time but differ in how we choose to spend it. In truth, it will take just one–forty-eighth of your whole day to exercise for thirty minutes. Most people waste a lot more time than that on unproductive activities like watching TV or surfing the Internet.

Saying, "I don't have enough time to exercise," will block your ability to recognize opportunities for physical activity because your brain doesn't believe they exist. On the other hand, you probably make time for grooming routines like bathing, putting on makeup, and shaving because you decide to do so.

I make time for my health and well-being is an abundance thought. You have time for the things that are the most important to you. Being physically active is more important for your health and well-being than most of the other things you think must get done each day. If you're too busy for exercise, you're just too busy! The key is to give exercise the priority it deserves. You could ask your partner to watch your kids for an hour so you can go to the YMCA, or you could walk with a friend you don't get to spend enough time with.

If it's easier or more convenient for you, breaking your exercise sessions into smaller chunks throughout the day is just as beneficial as one longer session. You could do ten minutes in the morning, ten minutes after lunch, and ten minutes in the afternoon, and it would still "count."

Self-Defeating vs. Affirming

I don't have the energy becomes a self-fulfilling prophecy because if you don't exercise, you'll continue to have low energy.

Replace self-defeating thoughts with affirming ones like *I feel myself becoming healthier and more energetic each day.* Have you ever noticed that fit people seem to have more energy than others? It turns out that exercise increases your strength and stamina, and it helps you to sleep better so that you become more productive and feel great.

No matter how you feel before you start exercising, you'll probably feel better within just a few minutes. These good feelings usually last long after the exercise is finished too. So, even when you feel tired, commit to exercising for at least ten minutes. Promise yourself you can stop and try again another day if you still don't feel any better. If you don't want to do any more exercise, at least you did something. Most of the time, you'll feel so good that you'll want to continue.

Powerless vs. Powerful

I'll start exercising when I've lost some of this weight is a thought that, rather than helping you take charge of the situation, leaves you waiting for something to happen. If you don't exercise while you're losing weight you may lose valuable muscle. It can become gradually harder to lose weight, and almost impossible to keep it off.

Replace powerless thoughts with powerful thoughts like *I support my weight-loss efforts and metabolism with regular exercise.* Doing any kind of extra physical activity helps balance your calories. In addition, physical activity reduces cravings and curbs your appetite by raising your endorphin (feel-good chemicals) and serotonin levels (calm chemicals). Besides, cardiorespiratory exercise and strength training minimize your loss of lean body mass during weight loss, which prevents a decrease in your metabolism. Most important, exercise improves your health whether you lose weight or not.

Outdated Thinking vs. Forward Thinking

If your past experience with exercise led to severe discomfort or pain, there's a good chance you may have worked out at an intensity that was too great for your level of fitness at the time, leaving you thinking, *Exercise is too hard for me.*

But you can replace this outdated thinking with forward thinking: *I have more stamina, strength, and flexibility every day.* Physical activity doesn't have to be hard and hurt to be beneficial. It's important to find activities that are comfortable, convenient, and fun so that you'll stick with them. Even if you have physical limitations, it's always possible to find some way to increase your activity level. If you've been very inactive, start by increasing your lifestyle activity by taking your dog for walks or washing your windows; then work toward a regular exercise routine. You'll be amazed at how your body adapts to whatever challenges you give it.

Judgmental vs. Unconditional

I'm too embarrassed to be seen exercising. If you judge yourself harshly, you may assume that other people judge you in the same way. Ironically, most other people are so focused on themselves that they don't notice you anyway. Those who do will likely admire you for making an effort to take care of yourself.

Replace judgmental thoughts with unconditional thoughts like *I exercise to take care of me.* Find activities and places that make you feel comfortable so that you can focus on all the wonderful benefits. Remember, you're doing this for yourself—to feel better and become healthier.

Shaming vs. Accepting

I'm so out of shape, I don't even know where to start! is a shaming thought. There's no such thing as instant fitness. If you don't choose to start somewhere, don't be surprised when you're still out of shape months from now.

A more accepting thought is *I have to start somewhere!* If you choose to start this week by increasing your movement and physical activity little by little, you'll become leaner, stronger, more energetic, and healthier.

If you haven't been physically active at all, you may need to check with your doctor before starting. Once you've been medically cleared, you have to start somewhere, so start right where you are.

Black and White vs. Shades of Gray

I can't do what they recommend, so why bother? This is all-or-nothing, or black-and-white, thinking. The notion that you have to exercise for thirty to sixty minutes, four to five days a week, or not at all is another pendulum swinging from one extreme to the other.

I do what I can to become more fit and healthy is a less rigid thought. Increased activity throughout the day really adds up. Taking the stairs, walking a little faster, and working or playing more actively every day can accomplish this. Every bit of activity over your usual level counts, so be on the lookout for opportunities to "just do it."

Ineffective vs. Effective

I have a strenuous job, so I don't need to exercise when I get home is an ineffective thought. Your activity level, both at work and at home, definitely contributes to your overall health, but few jobs provide all the elements of a great fitness program.

A more effective thought is *I am building a great overall fitness plan for myself.* Your fitness program should include lifestyle activity, cardiorespiratory activity, strength training, and flexibility for blood glucose management, prevention of disease, optimal energy, and good health.

Perfectionistic vs. Realistic

I was doing pretty well until I got sick (or *busy*, or *company came*, or *I went on vacation*) is a perfectionistic thought. To quit your exercise program because you missed a day, a week, or even longer makes as much sense as eating the whole bag of cookies because you ate three. No person and no schedule are ever perfect, but thinking that you have to do it perfectly will derail you every time.

A more realistic thought is *I have a flexible, consistent exercise program*. To make physical activity part of your life, try to be as consistent but as flexible as possible. Many people have found that writing their exercise schedules on their calendars helps them stay on track. If they miss a session, they simply reschedule it, as they would any other important appointment.

Outwardly Focused vs. Inwardly Focused

I started exercising but quit because I wasn't seeing the weight loss I expected is outwardly focused thinking. You won't see a change on the scale if you lose a pound of fat and build a pound of muscle, but your metabolism and glucose levels may improve. When you focus on weight loss, you'll lose sight of the most important goal: living an active, fulfilling, and healthy life.

Substitute inwardly focused thoughts: *I feel so good when I move my body*. Fitness is a process, and whether you're losing weight or not, you're becoming healthier. Set goals based on the many other benefits of exercise, like keeping your blood glucose level in the target range, having the stamina to play with your grandchildren, and not feeling winded by just walking to the mailbox.

Critical vs. Gentle

I used to be so athletic in high school; now I'm just a fat, lazy bum! It's easy to measure yourself against what you used to be able to do, but that only leads to critical self-talk. When you set the bar too high, the fear of failure will prevent you from trying to jump.

A gentler thought is *I'm not trying to compete in sports; I just want to be healthy.* Think about what's most important to you now instead of focusing on what used to be. When you're gentle with yourself, you'll make a lot more progress.

Problem Oriented vs. Solution Focused

I can't exercise because it's too cold (or *hot*) *outside* is a problem-oriented thought. Waiting for the perfect weather before exercising rules out much of the year in most places. It makes more sense to have different activities for different seasons and moods.

A solution-focused thought is *I have a lot of options for staying active, even when circumstances aren't ideal.* Dress in layers and head out at the best time of day depending on the weather. If the weather just isn't cooperating, there are lots of options for exercising in a climate-controlled environment. Think about working out at home to a DVD, taking classes at a fitness studio, using a treadmill or a stationary bike, dancing, and walking at an indoor mall.

Are Your Thoughts on Your Side?

Effective thinking is a habit, and new habits take practice. Start thinking of yourself as an active, healthy person—and you'll become one. For example, when you think, *Exercise is boring,* practice replacing this thought with *Being active gives me the opportunity to relieve stress and feel better.* When you repeat encouraging thoughts frequently, you'll begin to notice more-positive feelings, more-effective behaviors, and more-powerful results.

All of this applies to other aspects of your life too, like eating, relationships, work, and finances. If you don't like your results in any area of your life, ask yourself what you were thinking first. What other negative thoughts, attitudes, and feelings do you have that might be limiting you? Imagine how having more realistic, positive, and powerful thoughts could lead to feelings and actions that give you the results you desire. Now that's good food for thought!

Live a Vibrant Life!

In the coming "Live" chapters, you'll learn strategies for developing a positive attitude and building your motivation to increase your lifestyle activity and exercise. You'll see how you can boost your metabolism, decrease insulin resistance, improve your glucose levels, increase your energy, and enhance your sense of well-being. We'll also explore ways for you to steadily and comfortably build your stamina, strength, and flexibility. Ultimately, the real purpose is to help you reconnect with your body and rediscover that being active allows you to live a healthier, vibrant life.

PART 2

Curiosity

Curiosity will conquer fear even more than bravery will.

—James Stephens

CHAPTER 5

Think:
When Do I Want to Eat?

This chapter is devoted to the "when" part of the mindful eating cycle, as in "When do I want to eat?" Noticing that you want to eat is a good reminder to become aware of what's happening in that moment.

From this awareness arises curiosity about what hunger feels like, where your blood glucose level is at that moment, what could be causing the desire to eat if you *aren't* hungry, and what happens depending on how you decide to respond. Awareness and curiosity will also help you recognize how eating, physical activity, diabetes medications, and other factors influence your blood glucose.

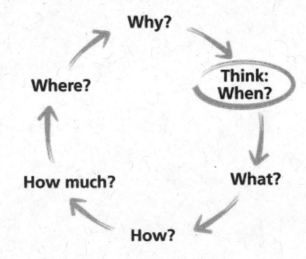

Figure 5.1

How Hunger Helps

You were born knowing exactly when and how much to eat. Hunger is your body's way of communicating that you need fuel. Reconnecting with your hunger signals helps you manage your diabetes. Here's how:

- You'll eat less food when you eat to satisfy physical hunger than when you eat to satisfy other needs. Think about it. If you aren't hungry when you start eating, how do you know when to stop?

- Food actually tastes better when you're physically hungry. Hunger really is the best seasoning—so you eat less but enjoy your food more.

- You're more likely to choose foods that nourish you. If you aren't hungry but are eating because you are sad, mad, or glad, what kinds of foods do you want? Isn't that when you're more likely to want chocolate, cookies, chips, or other comfort foods?

- You'll feel more satisfied, because food is great for taking care of hunger but not so great for addressing boredom, stress, or other triggers.

- When you notice that you're hungry before you get too hungry, you're less likely to overeat.

- There is overlap among the symptoms of hunger, low blood glucose, and high blood glucose. Learning to recognize the differences will help you respond appropriately to each of them.

- Noticing and responding to hunger before the symptoms are extreme can prevent hypoglycemia if you're on medication that can cause it.

What Gets in the Way?

Noticing when you're hungry may sound easy enough, but internal and external influences may have caused your natural system of regulating your food intake to go haywire.

Perhaps you think you're hungry all the time. Could you be misinterpreting other physical symptoms and sensations like thirst, fatigue, or high blood glucose? Do you confuse emotional or environmental triggers, cravings, and appetite with hunger?

Maybe you never feel hungry. Could it be that you eat so often in response to other triggers that your body never needs to tell you it needs more fuel? Perhaps you never get hungry because you've been told to eat on a schedule. Or maybe you have forgotten what hunger feels like, or get too busy or distracted to notice until the symptoms are really strong.

Recognizing Head Hunger

Whether or not you're aware of them yet, past experiences and associations affect how you eat now. Before we describe hunger, let's take a closer look at some of the causes of *head hunger*: triggers for eating when you're *not* physically hungry.

Physical Triggers

You can mistake some physical symptoms and sensations, like thirst, fatigue, or pain, for hunger. As we'll discuss later, *hyperglycemia* (high blood glucose) can also cause physical symptoms that resemble hunger at times.

Environmental Triggers

Have you ever suddenly felt like eating when you walked by doughnuts in the break room at work? It's common for people to confuse this sudden urge to eat with true hunger, but environmental situations often trigger head hunger whether your body needs food or not. These triggers develop when certain activities, people, or places are paired with eating so often that they become linked in your mind: one automatically goes with the other.

As Mark said in chapter 1, "Food has become the background music to our lives." Environmental triggers include mealtimes, holidays, advertisements, entertainment, social situations, friends and family members, restaurants, and even certain rooms in your house. The abundance of calorie-dense, appealing foods in increasingly larger portions has become a significant problem for people in many cultures. When you stop responding to these cues automatically, you can begin to change the way you think, feel, and react to them.

Emotional Triggers

Emotional connections to food are woven into the fabric of our social experience. From birth you were held and fed, you went to birthday parties for cake and ice cream, and you go out for dinner to celebrate a new job or a raise. Consider how common it is for people to use food as a way to bond, nurture, soothe, reward, love, celebrate, and create pleasure and excitement.

Emotions are also common triggers for overeating. People may eat to cope with stress, distract themselves from difficult emotions, or stuff down feelings they don't know how to express in a healthier manner.

It may not always be obvious to you when you're using food to cope with your feelings. You may think you're overeating just because it tastes good or because you lack willpower. Pausing to ask yourself, *Am I hungry?*, may reveal that the real reason you want the ice cream is to comfort or reward yourself for enduring a stressful day.

It isn't that using food to cope is wrong. But emotional eating becomes problematic when it's the primary way you deal with loneliness, boredom, anger, stress, anxiety, or depression. These feelings are a natural part of life. Since eating doesn't make them go away, your unmet needs can trigger overeating again and again. When you have diabetes, this method of coping leads to another problem: high blood glucose.

The way to break out of this pattern is to try to understand why you want to eat when you aren't physically hungry. When you identify the emotions that trigger the urge to eat, you have the option to seek other ways to comfort, nurture, calm, and distract yourself without turning to food. Of course, this is easier said than done! Seek out additional resources, like Michelle's previous book *Eat What You Love, Love What You Eat: How to Break Your Eat-Repent-Repeat Cycle*, if you need help.

Diabetes-Related Triggers

When you have diabetes, the idea of using hunger to guide your eating may seem puzzling, scary, or even ridiculous. This is common and understandable if you've been told you have to eat on a schedule. Maybe you've heard about hypoglycemia (low blood glucose) but aren't sure what causes it, so you've developed the habit of eating "just in case." Or perhaps you've had an episode of hypoglycemia in the past and eat to prevent yourself from ever having another one. Uncertainty, fear, and past experience may prevent you from using all of the information available to you in the present moment.

If you've struggled with your weight in the past, you may feel that you can't trust yourself to eat what you need. If you've been on restrictive diets, you may be familiar with the feelings of deprivation, cravings, overeating, and guilt that often result. Trying to follow a rigid diet because you have diabetes can have a similar effect.

Mindfulness helps you become aware of these other physical, environmental, and emotional cues for eating. You'll notice that *wanting* to eat isn't the same as *needing* to eat. Learning more about hunger and its relationship to blood glucose in this chapter will enable you to choose how to respond to a situation rather than to simply react out of habit.

Trust Your Body Wisdom

Can people who are out of touch with their hunger signals begin to recognize and, once again, use hunger to guide their intake? Definitely! Hunger is a natural, innate tool, and you can relearn the skills for using it effectively. By reconnecting with your instinctive signals, you can better manage your food intake and blood glucose levels without obsessing over every bite of food you put in your mouth—*even* if you have diabetes.

A remarkably simple but powerful way to become more aware of your body's cues is to ask yourself, *Am I hungry?*, whenever you want to eat. This important question will help you distinguish between an urge to eat caused by the physical need for food and an urge to eat caused by other physical, environmental, and emotional triggers.

What Does Hunger Feel Like?

Before reading ahead, stop and think for a moment. How do you know when you're hungry? What does it feel like? What are all the signs your body provides to let you know when you need to eat? Do you recognize any of these common hunger symptoms?

- Hunger pangs

- Growling or grumbling in the stomach

- An empty or hollow feeling

- Gnawing

- A slightly queasy feeling

- Weakness or loss of energy

- Trouble concentrating

- Difficulty making decisions

- Irritability or crankiness

- A slight headache

- Light-headedness

- Shakiness

- Feeling that you must eat as soon as possible

What Causes Hunger?

What do all these symptoms of hunger have in common? They are physical. They're not thoughts, feelings, or cravings. To become more aware of these physical sensations, it helps to understand what causes them. (We'll focus on normal hunger and fullness first, and we'll discuss hypoglycemia and hyperglycemia later.)

Hunger symptoms are caused by a combination of your stomach's emptiness or fullness, your body's need for energy, and various hormones and other substances in your body. We'll focus on your stomach and blood glucose, since they cause the most recognizable symptoms.

Your stomach is composed of muscle-like tissue that squeezes food to break it apart, mix it with digestive enzymes, and move it into your intestines. When your stomach is empty, its muscular walls begin to contract, causing the growling or rumbling you feel or hear when you're hungry. You may also experience an empty or hollow feeling. Since the stomach produces small amounts of digestive acids even when there's no food there, some people get sensations of gnawing or queasiness.

At the same time, you may identify symptoms of your blood glucose dropping. Your body and brain primarily use glucose from your bloodstream for energy. As your blood glucose falls, you may notice your energy level begin to dip and find it harder to concentrate and make decisions. When you're extremely hungry, you might develop a headache or feel light-headed and shaky.

Hunger and dropping blood glucose can also trigger changes in thoughts and mood. Many people become irritable, impatient, cranky, or short tempered when they're hungry. They may also have a diminished ability to think clearly about eating and other necessary decisions when they're really hungry.

Hunger is initially subtle and becomes stronger until you reach a point when you feel you absolutely must eat. If you wait any longer, you simply won't care what you eat as long as you get something into your stomach. That's why waiting to eat until you feel ravenous often leads to mindless food choices and overeating, which creates a cycle of high and low blood glucose levels that leaves you feeling drained, frustrated, and out of control.

Strategies: Body-Mind-Heart Scan

When you learn a new skill, it helps to have a strategy. Throughout this book, we'll provide specific strategies to help you build the skills you need to eat mindfully. Try not to focus on whether you are doing them "right." Instead, practice until they become natural for you.

An important mindfulness skill is awareness of your physical sensations, thoughts, and feelings. Doing a body-mind-heart scan will allow you to pause and observe what's going on inside right then. This skill is particularly useful when you feel like eating but aren't sure whether it's from physical hunger or head hunger. When you pause to become fully present and mindful, you can better identify your true needs.

1. **Pause:** If possible, close your eyes for a moment. Take a few deep breaths and calm yourself. Be aware that being near food or thinking about eating might cause you to feel excited or anxious, making it more difficult to identify the signs of hunger. By taking a few calming breaths first, you'll reconnect your body and mind, making it easier to focus on important sensations and feelings.

2. **Body:** In your mind's eye, scan your body from head to toe. What physical sensations are you aware of? Are you thirsty or tired? Are you aware of any tension, discomfort, or pain? Does your body feel good? Ask yourself, *Am I hungry?*, and connect with your body by placing your hand on your upper abdomen, just below your rib cage. Picture your stomach. Think of a balloon and try to imagine how full it is. When empty, it's about the size of your fist and can stretch several times that size when full. Are there pangs or gnawing sensations? Is there any growling or rumbling? Does your stomach feel empty, full, or even stuffed? Or perhaps you don't feel your stomach at all. Notice other physical sensations. Do you feel edgy, light-headed, or weak? Are these signals coming from hunger, low blood glucose, or something else? This is a great opportunity to become mindful of your body's signals and reconnect with your inner self.

3. **Mind:** Without judgment, notice what you are thinking. Quite often, your thoughts will give you clues about whether or not you're hungry. If you find yourself rationalizing or justifying, *It's been three hours since lunch, so I should be hungry,* you may be looking for an excuse to eat. If you have any doubts about whether you're hungry, you probably aren't.

4. **Heart:** What emotions are you experiencing now? What feelings are you aware of? When you become aware of your emotions, you can better see whether they affect your desire to eat—and even what or how much you want to eat.

What Happens When You Eat?

When you eat, hunger subsides as food fills your stomach and is broken down by your digestive system to be absorbed and used by your body. Depending on what you ate, the food is broken into glucose (from carbohydrates), fatty acids (from fats), amino acids (from proteins), and micronutrients, like vitamins and minerals. The type of food and how much you eat determine how high your blood glucose rises and how long it stays elevated. As you learned in chapter 2, under normal circumstances, your body releases insulin from your pancreas in response to the presence of glucose. Insulin acts like a key to unlock the cells to let energy enter in the form of glucose. Your body uses the energy for its activities and stores any extra fuel as body fat until it's needed. When your stomach is empty again and your blood glucose levels decrease, your body is ready to process more fuel, and the eating cycle repeats itself.

How Hungry Are You?

The Hunger and Fullness Scale is a useful tool for assessing your hunger and fullness levels before, during, and after eating. It will help you identify hunger cues, observe how different types and amounts of food affect you, and recognize the relationship between how you feel and your blood glucose level. This scale is not intended to set rules about when or what you should eat; rather, it helps you develop a greater awareness of your body's subtle signals.

The Hunger and Fullness Scale

The Hunger and Fullness Scale ranges from 1 to 10, with level 1 representing ravenous—you're so hungry you could eat this book—and level 10 meaning you're so full that you're in pain and feel sick. Remember, smaller numbers equal a smaller stomach, and larger numbers mean a larger stomach. In the middle of the scale is level 5, which means being satisfied and comfortable. At 5, you cannot feel your stomach at all. It's neither empty nor full; it isn't growling and doesn't feel stretched.

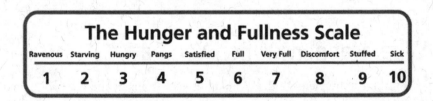

The Hunger and Fullness Scale

Ravenous	Starving	Hungry	Pangs	Satisfied	Full	Very Full	Discomfort	Stuffed	Sick
1	2	3	4	5	6	7	8	9	10

Figure 5.2

It may be challenging at first to label your hunger and fullness levels with numbers, but as you practice, it becomes second nature. Here are some descriptions to help you use the numbers to describe your levels of hunger and fullness.

1. *Ravenous:* Too hungry to care what you eat. This is a high-risk time for overeating. (If you are on glucose-lowering medications, this may be a sign of impending hypoglycemia. Check your blood glucose if possible.)

2. *Starving:* You feel you must eat *now!* Your blood glucose is likely dropping.

3. *Hungry:* Eating would be pleasurable, but you can wait longer.

4. *Pangs:* You're slightly hungry; you notice your first thoughts of food.

5. *Satisfied:* You're content and comfortable. You're neither hungry nor full; you can't feel your stomach at all.

6. *Full:* You can feel the food in your stomach.

7. *Very full:* Your stomach feels stretched, and you feel sleepy and sluggish.

8. *Discomfort:* Your stomach is too full, and you wish you hadn't eaten so much.

9. *Stuffed:* Your clothes feel very tight, and you're very uncomfortable.

10. *Sick:* You feel sick, in pain, or both.

It helps to develop a good mental picture of what's happening to your stomach at these different levels of hunger and fullness. Make a fist with your right hand. When your stomach is completely empty, it's about that size. This is level 1. One or two handfuls of food will take you from level 1 to level 5. It's surprising, isn't it, when you think about how large most serving sizes are? When you don't overfill your stomach, you feel light and comfortable after eating. Additionally, you are less likely to have a blood glucose level above your target when you don't overfill your stomach.

Another way to picture your stomach is to think of a balloon. When it's empty, you're at level 1. When you blow that first puff of air into the balloon, it fills out gently and takes its shape. That's level 5. As you take a deep breath and force more air into a balloon, its elastic walls begin to stretch and expand.

These are levels 6 through 10. Your stomach can stretch to 10 to hold excess food, so numbers over 5 indicate how stretched or uncomfortable your stomach feels. Most of us have eaten so much at one time or another that we've said, "If I eat one more bite, I'll pop!" When you feel this way, you're at level 10. We'll talk more about fullness in chapter 17.

Of course, changes in blood glucose levels, energy levels, moods, and substances in the bloodstream resulting from the digestive process also affect hunger and fullness signals. These other clues help communicate how hungry or full you are. You'll find it helpful to log your hunger and fullness levels alongside your blood glucose levels to see how they are related.

When Is the Best Time to Eat?

Your hunger and fullness levels usually mimic the rise and fall of your blood glucose, so you can use the Hunger and Fullness Scale to begin to fine-tune your eating patterns for optimal energy and glucose control. Starting in the middle, let's work our way down the scale.

Level 5 or higher. If you're at level 5 or above and want to eat or keep eating, you know that something other than hunger triggered this urge. This is an opportunity to learn more about yourself and how you respond to your environment and emotions.

Level 4. When your hunger level is at 4, you're slightly hungry and starting to think about eating. You can begin to plan for it by making sure time and food will be available when you're ready to eat. There will be times when you'll want to eat even though you're only slightly hungry, for example, at a mealtime or when you won't have another opportunity to eat later. Just keep in mind that if you're only a little hungry, you need only a little food.

Level 3 or 2. The ideal time to begin eating is when you reach level 3 or 2. At this point you're significantly hungry, so food will be pleasurable and satisfying. Eating at this point also prevents a low blood glucose reaction if you're on medications that put you at risk for hypoglycemia, as we'll explore next. It's important to plan meals ahead of time and to be prepared to respond to hunger even when it's not a conventional mealtime. Keep nutritious foods on hand—in your office, purse, briefcase, car, gym bag, carry-on—to eat when you're hungry.

Level 1. If you put off eating or don't notice that you're hungry until you're famished or hypoglycemic, you may not think as clearly or make mindful decisions about what to eat. When you're at level 1, you're more likely to eat anything you can get your hands on and to eat too quickly to notice when you've had enough. That's why you can easily go from starving to stuffed. If you are at risk for hypoglycemia, it's especially important to monitor your hunger symptoms, blood glucose levels, or both so you can respond rapidly and appropriately.

How Does Diabetes Affect Hunger?

Emerging research shows that having diabetes can affect your perception of hunger, although the mechanism is not completely understood yet (Kiyici et al. 2009; Kusaka et al. 2008; Bojanowska and Nowak 2007; Pinelli et al. 2011). In addition, with diabetes, your hunger symptoms may overlap with the symptoms of both *hyper*glycemia (high blood glucose) and *hypo*glycemia (low blood glucose) (Ciampolini and Biachi 2006; Ciampolini, Lovell-Smith, and Sifone 2010; Ciampolini et al. 2010). How could that be?

Overlap Between Hunger, Hypoglycemia, and Hyperglycemia

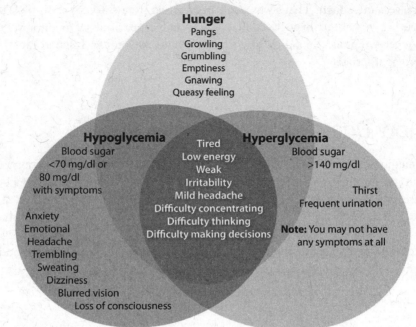

Figure 5.3

Hyperglycemia

As you learned in chapter 2, with diabetes you can have plenty of glucose in the bloodstream (hyperglycemia), but it can't get into the cells. Since the cells aren't getting the fuel they need, they are starving. Therefore, you may feel tired, drained, or sad and experience low energy or difficulty thinking. It's easy to see why high blood glucose can be confused with hunger, just as Gloria realized:

I didn't know why I was hungry all the time, but I kept hoping that if I ate something, I'd have more energy. It didn't work, and instead I just kept gaining weight. After I was diagnosed with diabetes, I started to make some changes to my diet and have noticed that my energy level is improving.

Hypoglycemia

"Hypoglycemia" literally means low blood glucose and is defined as a blood glucose of less than 70 mg/dL. You'll learn about blood glucose testing in the next chapter and more about hypoglycemia in chapter 18.

It's important to know that having diabetes does not cause hypoglycemia. However, some of the medications used to treat diabetes lower your blood glucose and, therefore, can cause hypoglycemia, especially if a meal is missed or delayed, or if there is more activity than usual. Ask your health care professional if your medication can cause hypoglycemia.

The symptoms of hypoglycemia can vary and may include hunger, difficulty concentrating, headache, trembling, shaking, irritability or anger, pale skin, sweats, dizziness, anxiety, irrational behavior, confusion, and unconsciousness.

Hunger is often the first symptom of a decrease in your blood glucose, and it simply indicates that it's time to eat. As your blood glucose levels decrease, symptoms of hypoglycemia can make it difficult to continue your current activity because you don't feel well. Severe hypoglycemia can become very serious and must be recognized and treated (see chapter 18). If you are at risk for hypoglycemia, add a zero to the left side of your Hunger and Fullness Scale to remind you to watch for symptoms that require immediate action.

Hunger & Fullness with Hypoglycemia

Hypo-glycemia	Ravenous	Starving	Hungry	Pangs	Satisfied	Full	Very Full	Discomfort	Stuffed	Sick
0	1	2	3	4	5	6	7	8	9	10

Figure 5.4

If your blood glucose falls below 70 mg/dL, you need to consume 15 to 20 grams of carbohydrate, such as 4 ounces of juice or soda (not diet soda), six saltine crackers, an appropriate number of glucose tablets, glucose gel, or whatever your health care provider advises. Recheck your blood glucose in 15 minutes to make sure it is 70 mg/dL or above. If it's still low, eat another serving of 15 grams of carbohydrate and recheck in 15 minutes. If you can't consume carbohydrate by mouth, 911 should be called immediately. Carry glucose tablets or gel with you, wear a medical bracelet, and be sure that others you spend time with are aware of emergency instructions too.

Your Hunger Rhythms

Although your body may not work perfectly when you have diabetes, mindful eating helps increase your awareness of what's going on so you can make decisions that support you.

Paul told us how becoming mindful of his hunger levels helped stabilize his blood glucose and improve his diabetes:

After I started checking my blood glucose, I became more interested in what causes it to change. One thing I noticed was that when I was too hungry, I overate, so, of course, my blood sugar spiked. I started paying attention to my hunger so I could eat before it got out of hand. This was a huge shift for me because I was no longer going from one extreme to the other, which has made managing my diabetes so much easier.

Eating according to your hunger and fullness signals supplies a consistent fuel source and levels out your blood glucose. As a result, you'll experience fewer mood and energy swings and fewer low and high blood glucose levels. Along with the other strategies introduced in the coming chapters, you'll likely discover that you feel more physically *and* emotionally in charge of your diabetes when you eat this way.

CHAPTER 6

Care:
Glucose Monitoring

While your hunger symptoms help you determine when, what, and how much to eat, your glucose monitoring helps you see how your blood glucose is *affected* by when, what, and how much you eat—as well as other factors, like physical activity, stress, and medications. In this chapter, you'll see that viewing your blood glucose results with curiosity rather than fear and judgment can unlock many mysteries surrounding diabetes.

Fearless Blood Glucose Monitoring

If you've avoided consistent blood glucose testing in the past, ask yourself why. Perhaps you didn't understand the purpose or know what to do with the results. Maybe you thought it was too much trouble, too expensive, or too uncomfortable.

Another common reason people don't test is the fear that their blood glucose levels will be used as evidence of "cheating." There's an assumption that if your blood glucose is high, you did something wrong and should therefore feel guilty and ashamed. If this sounds familiar, maybe you didn't want to know the results because that might mean a change was necessary: *Why should I check my blood glucose? I'm going to eat the cake anyway!* or *I ate too much, so I already know it will be high.*

Whatever the reasons, when you don't check your blood glucose, you are missing an opportunity to learn. By approaching it with interest and curiosity rather than trepidation and judgment, you may even find that testing is fun—sort of like solving a puzzle. Okay, maybe "fun" is too strong a word, but relax a little and see what you discover!

How to Keep a Blood Glucose Log

When you look at the numbers, monitoring your glucose is a powerful tool to become aware of how various factors affect your blood glucose levels. This is an important shift toward taking charge of your health and reducing the stress associated with managing your diabetes.

A One-Week Experiment

If you are not checking your blood glucose regularly and are willing to give it a try, conduct a one-week experiment to see what you can learn. Here's a great way to get started:

1. Download the Fearless Blood Glucose Monitoring Log from www.mindfuleatinganddiabetes.com, use one your health care team provides, or explore blood glucose tracking tools to use on your computer or smart phone.

2. Test and record your blood glucose twice a day for the next seven days (a total of fourteen blood glucose tests).

3. Test your blood glucose before or two hours after a meal, or both. *Paired glucose testing*, which is blood glucose testing right before and two hours after eating, offers a lot of information, which we'll explore further later.

4. Also check your blood glucose when you think it might be low and when you think you may have eaten too much. Remember, the purpose is to help you learn, not to cause blame, shame, or guilt.

5. Jot down your hunger and fullness levels, as well as notes about other physical sensations, your meal, physical activity, and anything else you think might help you understand your blood glucose levels.

7-day Fearless Blood Glucose Monitoring Log

Directions: Test your blood glucose twice a day. Paired blood glucose tests—right before and two hours after eating—offer a lot of information. Circle your hunger and fullness (H & F) level before (B) and after (A) eating. Write down other notes like physical activity, what you ate, how you felt, questions, and so on.

Your Personal Target Blood Glucose: _____
Suggested: Fasting or before meals: 70–130 mg/dL; 2 hours after eating <180 mg/dL

Week 6/22	Meal:		Meal:		Meal:		Meal:	
Sun	Before	2 hrs after	Before	2 hrs after	Before	2 hrs after	Before	2 hrs after
	182	219						
Rate your H & F	B A 0 1 2 ③ 4 5 ⑥ 7 .8 9 10		0 1 2 3 4 5 6 7 8 9 10		0 1 2 3 4 5 6 7 8 9 10		0 1 2 3 4 5 6 7 8 9 10	
Notes	BKF: Cereal, milk, juice				Walked dog for 25 min			
Mon	Before	2 hrs after	Before	2 hrs after	Before	2 hrs after	Before	2 hrs after
			93	136				
Rate your H & F	0 1 2 3 4 5 6 7 8 9 10		B A 0 1 2 3 ④ 5 6 ⑦ 8 9 10		0 1 2 3 4 5 6 7 8 9 10		B A 0 1 2 3 4 ⑤ ⑥ 7 8 9 10	
Notes			Lunch: Turkey Sandwich, apple, carrots, water				Bored Ate 4 cookies	
Tues	Before	2 hrs after	Before	2 hrs after	Before	2 hrs after	Before	2 hrs after
					112	186		
Rate your H & F	0 1 2 3 4 5 6 7 8 9 10		0 1 2 3 4 5 6 7 8 9 10		B A 0 ① 2 3 4 5 6 7 ⑧ 9 10		0 1 2 3 4 5 6 7 8 9 10	
Notes	Walked dog for 30 minutes				Dinner: Stir fry veggies, 2 cups of rice, glass of wine			

Figure 6.1

On Target

Now let's take a look at your blood glucose log and try to interpret the testing to more fully understand your diabetes, beginning with figuring out how often your blood glucose levels are in the target range.

1. Here are the typical target blood glucose levels when you have type 2 diabetes; check with your health care provider to confirm that these are the right targets for you:

    Fasting (nothing to eat for eight hours) or before meals: 70 to 130 mg/dL

    Two hours after eating: <180 mg/dL

2. Review your log and circle all of the blood glucose readings that are within these target ranges.

3. Next count all the blood glucose tests you took. We suggested fourteen tests; it's fine if you tested a different number of times.

4. Divide the number of blood glucose levels that were in your target range by the total number of tests you took and multiply by 100. That is the percent of tests that are in target. For example, six tests in your target range divided by fourteen total tests means that 43 percent were on target.

5. Place an "X" over blood glucose levels that are less than 70 mg/ dL; these are episodes of hypoglycemia.

6. Count the number of episodes of hypoglycemia; call your health care provider if you have two or more episodes in one week.

As you review your blood glucose readings, be aware of any judgment that arises and try to let it go. It isn't realistic to expect 100 percent of your blood glucose levels to be in your target range (Brewer et al. 1998). Instead, use the percentage of blood glucose measurements that are on target to help you monitor the effectiveness of changes to your diet, physical activity, and medication.

A Case for Curiosity

Using your powers of observation and curiosity, see if you can begin to interpret the results of your experiment. Look for patterns or trends that seem predictable. Make guesses about how your glucose numbers, eating, activity levels, and feelings are related. Here are some examples of questions you might ask yourself:

- *Do I have any feelings of guilt, blame, shame, or fear about blood glucose levels that are out of my target range?*

- *What do I notice about my blood glucose in the morning before I eat? What percentage is in my target range? What percentage is out of my target range?*

- *Without judgment, shame, blame, or guilt, do I have any guesses about why that happened?*

- *What do I notice about my after-meal blood glucose readings? What percentage is in my target range? What percentage is out of my target range?*

- *Without judgment, shame, blame, or guilt, what are my guesses about why that happened?*

- *Do I see any changes when I'm active or exercising?*

- *How does physical activity affect me?*

- *How do I feel physically this week? Am I sleepy, alert, weak, strong, hungry, tired, or anything else?*

- *How do I feel emotionally this week?*

- *How are these emotional and physical feelings related to my diabetes, blood glucose, eating, physical activity, or other variables?*

Always take your blood glucose log with you to appointments. Your memory only has to be as sharp as a pencil or as close as your computer! By keeping a detailed blood glucose log, you can show your health care team how your diabetes treatments—diet, activity, and medications—are working and ask for their help in understanding these variables.

Checking your blood glucose regularly, becoming curious, looking for patterns, and making observations are big steps toward taking charge of your diabetes.

Strategies: What Does Your Blood Glucose Feel Like?

The body-mind-heart scan helps you tune in to subtle cues that are commonly missed when you are distracted or busy. Using blood glucose testing as an additional piece of information, see if you can become more aware of what different blood glucose levels feel like. This is particularly important if you are at risk for hypoglycemia since low blood glucose reactions rarely come at a good time. Most reactions occur when you are busy doing other things—playing, shopping, working, or sleeping—because the early signs of dropping blood glucose levels are ignored or mistaken for something else, or simply go unnoticed.

Become aware. For the next week, do a brief body-mind-heart scan *before* you test your blood glucose. Identify your hunger and fullness number, as well as any other physical sensations, thoughts, and feelings. Based on what you notice, estimate what your blood glucose might be.

Gather information. Test your blood glucose and write it down in your log. If you forgot to do a body-mind-heart scan beforehand, do it after your test. Just be aware that knowing the number can cloud or influence what you notice during your scan.

Be nonjudgmental. There are no wrong numbers—just information to help you and your health care team manage this disease more effectively. The impulse to think of a blood glucose number as "good" or "bad" often leads to thoughts that *you* are "good" if your blood glucose is "good" and "bad" if your blood glucose is "bad." Over time, such thinking drains you of the energy needed to care for your diabetes. Remember, your self-worth does *not* depend on your blood glucose.

Be curious. Did your reading make sense to you? Did you think, *Wow! I didn't think it would be that!* Ask yourself, *Do I feel any different when my blood glucose is above or below target? Were there any signs or clues that my blood glucose was low or dropping?* Here are some examples of what others noted:

Norman: "When my blood glucose is really high, I feel empty, like someone pulled the plug and all my energy left me."

Liz: "My eyelid twitches when my blood glucose is low."

Bob: "When my blood sugar is high, I feel funny, like I'm forgetting something."

Jen: "My head gets itchy when my blood glucose is high."

Joe: "I don't feel anything until my low blood sugar hits! I know I have to stop what I'm doing and treat it because if I don't, things just get worse."

Notice patterns. Take a moment to consider and record any possible reasons for your blood glucose reading in your log. Include information about your hunger and fullness levels; when, what, and how much you ate; and details about illnesses, physical activity, and other circumstances. Taking the time to write a quick note is better than relying on your memory later.

How Does Eating Affect My Blood Sugar?

It's important to see your glucose test results as clues that help you solve the mystery of how eating affects your diabetes. Paired glucose testing—blood glucose tests right before and two hours after eating—can help you learn more about your diabetes. In short, if your blood glucose is only elevated two hours after eating, your diet is probably contributing in some way. Before you think, *Oh no, I blew it!*, remember that eating is *supposed* to cause your blood glucose to rise. Resist blame, guilt, and restriction. Instead, explore possible connections between what you ate and what happens to your blood glucose. In the following chapters, we'll discuss how physical activity, medications, and the macronutrients—carbohydrate (sugar, starch, and fiber), protein, and fat—affect your blood glucose, but for now, use the power of awareness and curiosity to look for patterns.

CHAPTER 7

Nourish:
Mindful Meal Planning

A dmittedly, nutrition information can be confusing: Are potatoes vegetables or starches? Are nuts fats or proteins? Are kidney beans carbohydrates or protein? (All are both.)

If you sometimes feel overwhelmed by it all, you're not alone! Our goal is to teach you what you need to know about nutrition to manage your blood glucose and keep yourself healthy. Simultaneously, we want to give you a flexible approach to eating that is enjoyable and sustainable.

All Foods Fit

We firmly believe in an all-foods-fit approach to healthy eating—even when you have prediabetes or diabetes. Donna provides a good example of why:

When I learned I had prediabetes, I panicked. I had watched my mother lose her eyesight and her independence as a result of her diabetes, so I wasn't going to let that happen to me. My doctor said I needed to lose weight, so I started a low-carb diet. It was easy at first since the rule was that I could eat as much as I wanted as long as it wasn't a carb. I got bored with eating the same things all the time, so I ate less and lost eight pounds. I really started missing my bread, cereal, pasta, fruit, and especially chocolate—and I just didn't feel great. Besides, aren't whole grains and fresh fruits supposed to be good for you? I just couldn't stay motivated to stick with it and quickly gained back everything I'd lost—except my self-esteem!

While some foods are more nutrient rich than others, all foods can fit into balanced eating. We'll use three simple but essential principles for effectively implementing this all-foods-fit approach to eating: balance, variety, and moderation.

Principle 1: Balance. Balancing your energy intake with your energy output is important for glucose and weight management. Balancing eating for nourishment with eating for enjoyment is important for sustainable lifestyle change. Donna's low-carbohydrate diet left her feeling out of balance.

Principle 2: Variety. Variety refers to eating an assortment of foods. As Donna discovered, eating the same foods all the time leads to monotony. Not only was it boring, but it also wasn't meeting all of her nutritional requirements. It's important to eat from all of the food groups and to eat a variety of foods within each group, since no single food has everything you need. Variety in eating promotes overall health and enjoyment.

Principle 3: Moderation. Moderation refers to how much and how often you eat certain things. Mindfulness will help you recognize when you've had enough. When your goal is to feel good after eating, you're more likely to eat in moderation. As you become more tuned in to your body's signals and the experience of eating, you're also more likely to enjoy fresh, wholesome foods and choose less-healthful foods in moderation.

Planning Your Plate

In later "Nourish" chapters, you'll learn more about how the macronutrients—carbohydrate, fat, and protein—affect your blood glucose and your health. However, we don't consume isolated *nutrients*—we eat *food*. Therefore, a more practical way to think about nutrition is to look at the food on your plate. The United States Department of Agriculture (USDA) introduced "My Plate" to help people eat a more healthful diet by visualizing the meal as different food groups. The website, www.choosemyplate.gov, has a lot of helpful information about using this method, including examples of foods in each group. Since "My Plate" was designed for the general population, we've made changes to make it more helpful for people with diabetes.

Love What You Eat with Diabetes Plate

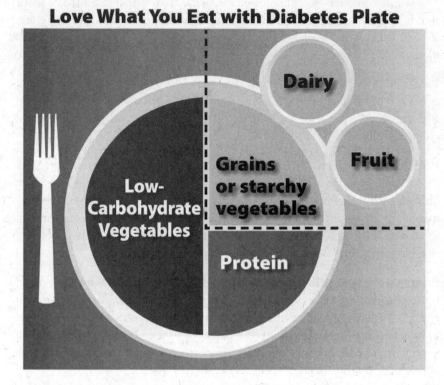

Figure 7.1

Start by picturing your meal and visually dividing your plate in half. Fill the left half of your plate with low-carbohydrate vegetables.

Divide the other half of your plate in half again and put lean protein in the bottom section and grains or starchy vegetables in the top section. To the right of that, add a serving of fruit and a serving of dairy. If you prefer, you can "save" your fruit or milk for a snack rather than have it with your meal.

Since most people don't eat vegetables for breakfast, picture your breakfast plate divided into four sections: grains, fruit, dairy, and protein.

We like the simplicity of the plate method because it gives you flexibility in planning your meals. When you have prediabetes or diabetes, there are a few other things to keep in mind to support your health. We'll cover the details in the later "Nourish" chapters, but here's a sneak preview.

Carbohydrates Count

As you learned in chapter 2, with diabetes, your body can't process glucose efficiently. Therefore, it's necessary to be mindful of the total amount of carbohydrate you eat at each meal or snack so that your carbohydrate intake doesn't exceed your body's ability to process the glucose. As you'll learn in chapter 11, the foods in the upper-right portion of the Love What You Eat with Diabetes Plate—grains and starchy vegetables, fruit, and dairy—contain approximately 15 grams of carbohydrate per serving, so you want to pay close attention to these choices when you have diabetes. On the other hand, non-starchy vegetables are low in carbohydrate, typically 5 grams or less per serving. Visualizing your plate allows you to easily determine how to adjust your meal or snack for optimal glucose management.

Fat Matters

Fat matters, even though you don't see it on this picture of a plate. In fact, most of the time, you won't see it on your actual plate either! That's because it often hides in snack foods, animal products, and dressings and sauces and is used in frying, sautéing, and baking.

Fat slows down glucose absorption, increases satiety (satisfaction and fullness), and stabilizes blood sugar levels. The type of fat you eat is important for your health. Eating an excessive amount of solid fats increases your risk of heart disease, whereas replacing solid fats with oils decreases this risk. Since having diabetes puts you at increased risk for heart disease, you'll want to be mindful about the type and amount of fat you eat. In chapter 15 you'll learn more about the connection between solid fats and heart disease.

Protein Power

Protein increases satiety (fullness and satisfaction), so you may eat less and feel satisfied longer. Chapter 19 explores protein as a powerful part of a balanced plate.

What about Snacks, Desserts and Alcohol?

People with diabetes often ask if they *should* eat snacks and whether they *can* have desserts or alcohol. The mindful eating cycle puts *you* in charge of these decisions.

Snacks Are Mini Meals

People with diabetes don't necessarily need snacks. It's helpful to think of snacks as mini meals that provide fuel and nutrients. When deciding whether to have a snack, ask, *Am I hungry?*, and determine how hungry you are to help you decide whether your body needs additional fuel and if so, how much. It is also helpful to consider when you might eat again, especially if you are at risk for hypoglycemia.

Desserts and Sweets

There's a common misconception that eating sugar causes diabetes and that people with diabetes aren't allowed to eat sugar. It's true that sugar is a carbohydrate, so it will raise your glucose level—all carbohydrates do. That doesn't make sugar "bad" and make you bad for liking it! In fact, telling yourself you can't have it can lead to feelings of deprivation, cravings, overeating, and guilt: the eat-repent-repeat cycle that wreaks havoc with your blood glucose.

A more helpful approach is to acknowledge that the primary purpose of eating desserts and sweets is pleasure, so it doesn't make sense to ruin the experience with guilt, thoughts of failure, or feeling too full. Instead, if you really like them, fit sweets and desserts into your diet in moderation by including their carbohydrate content in your total for that snack or meal. Chapter 11 has more on how to do that.

Alcohol

In people with diabetes, light to moderate alcohol intake (one to two drinks per day) is associated with a decreased risk of cardiovascular disease

(ADA 2008). However, the benefits do not outweigh the risks in people with a history of alcohol abuse or dependence, liver disease, pancreatitis, advanced neuropathy, or severe hypertriglyceridemia. If you choose to use alcohol, use moderation (less than one drink per day for adult women and less than two drinks per day for adult men). Alcohol should be consumed with food to reduce risk of nighttime low blood glucose for those at risk. Keep in mind that alcoholic beverages made with mixers that contain carbohydrates will raise blood glucose levels.

Using Nutrition Labels

Detailed nutrition labels, called "Nutrition Facts," provide information about portion size, nutrient content, ingredients, and other details. To learn how to read a nutrition label, visit www.diabetesandmindfuleating.com/resources .html. There are two important things to keep in mind: First, use the nutrition label to educate yourself about the nutrient content of food, not to label food as "good" or "bad." Second, although a nutrition label has a lot of information, don't let it overwhelm you. Instead focus on the key information you're interested in.

Remember, there's no right or wrong food to eat. The point of reading labels is to educate yourself about what your food choices contain. To learn more about nutrition information, visit websites such as www.eatright.org, www.diabetes.org, or www.choosemyplate.gov.

You're in Charge

Continue to check in with yourself as you read this book and experiment with the nutrition concepts you are learning. When necessary, remind yourself that nutrition information is used most effectively as a tool, not a weapon. Being in charge gives you the flexibility to select foods that will be most satisfying to you while keeping your blood glucose levels in the target range. Awareness of the nutrient content of your food will help you make decisions about balance, variety, and moderation. Other tools, including nutrition labels and websites like www.eatright.org, can also help you learn more about the food you eat. Here's what Michael learned from planning his meal using the plate method.

I always start planning my meal by choosing my non-starchy vegetables first. I like to fill half my plate with veggies like salad, broccoli, green beans, or asparagus. I noticed that by focusing on eating more vegetables, I didn't miss the large portions of potatoes and bread I used to eat. Even when I make pasta, it's mostly vegetables: sautéed onions, mushrooms, peppers, and tomatoes over whole-grain pasta with a diced chicken breast—yum! Who knew balanced eating could be so good!

With awareness of nutrition and meal planning techniques, you can design flexible meals and snacks that are nourishing and satisfying and that help you keep your blood glucose in the target range.

CHAPTER 8

Live:
Exercise Is the Best Medicine

J ust as you were born with the instinctive ability to eat to meet your body's needs, you were born to move. In the distant past, movement was critical for survival. Today, modern society has ways to do almost everything more efficiently, automatically, and effortlessly. While these conveniences may save time, they also save energy—your energy.

The result? Increased body fat, decreased muscle mass, and weight gain—all feeding into the insulin resistance that underlies type 2 diabetes. Further, less movement and a low level of physical activity result in decreased fitness, so you may not have the stamina, flexibility, or strength to live your life to the fullest.

Mindfulness increases your awareness of what your body wants and needs to feel and function at its best. As you begin to move more, you'll discover improved blood glucose levels and increased energy, function, and vitality. As you develop a fitness program that is enjoyable and suits your personality, you'll nurture a positive, self-perpetuating cycle that improves your diabetes and your life.

Mastering Your Metabolism

Understanding your metabolism and how it works will help you see why physical activity makes such a difference.

What Is Metabolism Anyway?

The word "metabolism" is thrown around a lot these days. People often complain about having a slow or sluggish metabolism. Many products promise to boost your metabolism. But what *is* metabolism anyway? In a nutshell, metabolism simply refers to the amount of fuel or energy your body burns each day, pictured here as a fuel can. How you live your life determines your metabolism; it's *where* you invest your energy in the mindful eating cycle (review figure 1.1).

Metabolism

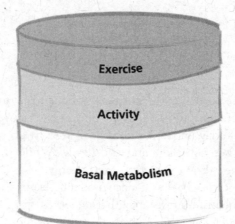

Figure 8.1

Your Basal Metabolism

Your basal metabolism is the number of calories your body needs to support your basic bodily functions. These vital functions include your heartbeat, breathing, brain function, and numerous other important but invisible activities going on inside of you at all times. Even eating, digesting, and processing food contribute to your metabolism.

In fact, every cell in your body is like a tiny engine that burns fuel continuously in the process of doing its job. These tiny engines never shut off—at least while you're alive. Even when you're sleeping or sitting still, your body's cells are still actively working just to keep you alive. It's just like your car: when the engine is running, it's burning fuel—even if it's just sitting in the driveway.

Boost Your Metabolism with Activity and Exercise

Your body's workload and, therefore, fuel needs increase with any type of activity above your basal metabolic level. For instance, your lung cells must work to take in oxygen and release carbon dioxide, but they work harder when you're walking than when you're sitting in a chair.

Everything you do throughout your day-to-day existence requires fuel, from brushing your teeth and taking a shower, to walking around your home or office. You're burning fuel right now, just reading this book. Of course, some activities require more fuel than others; the more you demand from your body, the more fuel each tiny cell burns while doing its job. A few added steps here and there and a little extra effort during routine work and play really add up.

Another great way to boost your metabolism is with regular exercise. Exercise not only burns more fuel while you're doing it but also increases the amount of fuel your cells burn for a while afterward. Obviously, a person who walks two miles a day requires more fuel and will be more fit than someone who doesn't exercise at all. As you'll see, the benefits of increasing your activity and adding exercise also extend beyond your metabolism. Forget all or nothing. Become more active by starting wherever you are, and increase gradually, step by step.

Fitness Rx: The FITT Formula

Use the FITT Formula to tailor a fitness program to your personal health needs, preferences, lifestyle, and goals. FITT stands for frequency, intensity, time, and type. Write your own fitness prescription:

Frequency: How often you will be active

Intensity: How much effort you'll use during activity

Time: How much time you'll invest in being active

Type: What kinds of activities you'll do

Every Little Bit Counts

Whether you're already active or not, even a few added steps here and there and a little extra effort during everyday tasks can add up to big benefits. Look at some simple ways to boost your lifestyle activities and underline the ideas you'll try. Remember to have fun!

At Leisure

- Play actively with your children or grandchildren. They love to play tag, ride bikes, or practice sports; don't be surprised if you strengthen your relationships too.

- Walk your dog, play fetch, or chase him around the backyard.

- Join an adult sports league, like softball, tennis, or bowling. Sign up for a walking, hiking, or jogging club.

- Walk the golf course and carry your own golf clubs instead of renting a cart.

- Take a swim to cool off and relax in the summer, or find an indoor pool in the winter.

- Reconnect at the end of the day with your partner or a friend on an evening walk.

- Instead of always eating out, choose dancing, bowling, or other active pursuits with friends. Plan a hike or a walking tour when you have out-of-town visitors.

At Home

- Housework, such as vacuuming, scrubbing floors, making beds, and washing windows, keeps both your home and your body in shape.

- Balance on one foot while you're cooking, washing dishes, or brushing your teeth.

- Instead of piling things at the bottom of the stairs, make a trip upstairs every chance you get.

- Do some floor exercises while you watch television, or stand up and stretch during the commercials. Even standing while you watch TV will burn more calories and build more muscle than just sitting.

- Tape your favorite daytime show to watch in the evening while you use a treadmill or stationary bike. Better yet, turn off the TV, turn on some music, and dance.

- Yard work, like mowing your lawn, weeding, and gardening, is great too.

- Wash your car, walk to the mailbox, get up to change the channels, and walk to the next room to talk instead of yelling.

- If the gym setting doesn't appeal to you, try an exercise video.

At Work

- Consider walking or riding your bike to work. Get off the bus or subway a stop or two early, or park in a distant parking space and walk the rest of the way.

- Use the stairs instead of the elevator; start with one flight, once a day, and gradually increase until you hardly use the elevator at all.

- Fidget. Fidgeting, like tapping your foot or bouncing your leg, requires energy.

- Stand and stretch, or walk around when you need a break.

- Take a walk during your lunch hour or use an onsite or nearby gym. Even better, ask a coworker to join you.

While Out

- Whenever possible, do your errands on foot. (They don't call it running errands for nothing!) Park your car in a central location and walk to all your destinations.

- Walk through the mall briskly. In fact, many malls open early so you can walk in a temperature-controlled environment; take a few laps and window-shop before the stores open.

- Take the stairs instead of the escalator or elevator.

- Stretch and tighten your muscles while waiting in lines or sitting at stoplights.

While Traveling

- Walk around the airport or conference center instead of sitting around waiting.

- See the local sights by foot or walk to attractions.

- Take advantage of the hotel's gym or the resort's exercise classes, or use the Internet for workouts you can do right in your hotel room.

- Use the stairs and walk to meetings and restaurants.

- Plan a vacation that includes lots of opportunities to rejuvenate your body and mind.

At Rest

- Stretch when you wake up and after sitting for a long time.

- Learn basic yoga or tai chi and practice daily.

- Try deep breathing exercises, relaxation techniques, and meditation.

- Give yourself time to relax at the end of the day.

- Get enough sleep so that you'll have plenty of energy for your more active lifestyle.

How Does Exercise Help Diabetes?

Your age, genes, activity level, weight, and body composition all influence insulin resistance. Of course, you can't change your age or genes, but the other three variables are affected by exercise. Let's take a look at how.

Physical Activity Lowers Your Blood Glucose

Since activity requires fuel, exercise can naturally lower your blood glucose, your body's primary source of fuel. A good rule of thumb is that you'll lower your glucose one point for every minute of mild to moderate exercise, up to about forty minutes (Sigal et al. 2004). In other words, forty minutes of exercise, like walking, yard work, or biking, will lower your blood glucose by forty points on average, *all* day! If you have prediabetes and walk for fifteen minutes during your lunch hour each day, you'll decrease your average blood glucose level by fifteen points for the rest of the day. This small, consistent change could actually prevent or delay the onset of diabetes. Exercise is truly the best prescription!

If your physical activity continues beyond thirty minutes, your body will also tap into the glucose stored as glycogen in your muscles and liver. Since it takes twenty-four to forty-eight hours to refill these glucose stores, your blood glucose levels are likely to be lower during that time (ibid.).

Exercise Improves Your Body Composition

Your body is composed of water, adipose tissue (better known as fat), and lean tissue, which is everything else (muscle, bone, hair, and other tissues). Exercise decreases fat and increases muscle mass, which decreases insulin resistance, thereby improving glucose regulation.

Muscle is called "metabolically active tissue" because the tiny engines of muscle cells burn more energy than less-active cells. That's why people say "a pound of muscle burns more calories each day than a pound of fat."

Muscle cells require not only more glucose to do their work but also more energy for maintenance. Whenever you do more than your body is accustomed to, your body builds additional muscle to accommodate the new workload. Building this new muscle tissue requires even more fuel. Of course, once you build additional muscle tissue, it takes more energy to maintain it. In short, by increasing your number of active cells, you increase the amount of glucose you burn. It's like a factory: as the number of workers increases, the productivity, or output, goes up.

Exercise: The Best Medicine

If you could bottle exercise, you'd have the closest thing there is to a wonder drug.

Brand Name: Exercise. Numerous effective generics available: aerobics, basketball, biking, body sculpting, dancing, hiking, housework, jogging, jumping rope, playing with children, racquetball, rowing, stretching, swimming, tennis, walking, walking the dog, weight lifting, working out, yard work, yoga, and many others.

Indications. Shown to be very effective for relief of fatigue, stress, low self-esteem, insomnia, boredom, and symptoms of depression and anxiety. May prevent, improve, or delay onset of the following conditions: prediabetes and diabetes, high blood pressure, high cholesterol, heart disease, some types of cancer, some forms of arthritis, fibromyalgia, premenstrual syndrome, constipation, addictions, overweight and obesity, and many other health problems.

Benefits. Increased energy and productivity, increased metabolism, weight loss, improved sense of well-being and appearance, better sleep patterns, improved sex life, improved appetite regulation, lower blood glucose, lower heart rate and blood pressure, higher HDL (good) cholesterol, improved blood glucose control, decreased medication dosages, and reduced risk of cancer.

Side effects. Patients report feeling stronger, healthier, energetic, and more youthful.

Precautions. Consult with your physician first, especially if you have any chronic medical conditions, heart problems, or unexplained symptoms. If you develop unexpected shortness of breath; chest, jaw, neck, or arm pain or pressure; rapid or irregular heart rate; light-headedness; pain; or any other unexplained symptoms, stop and seek immediate medical advice and attention.

Dosage. Start with small doses, taken most days of the week, and increase gradually as tolerance develops. Dosage may be adjusted, if necessary, to accommodate other responsibilities. Due to the many beneficial effects, consistent usage is very important. Choose among the numerous generic brands available and alternate brands as needed to improve overall level of fitness, and maintain interest and motivation.

Warning. Likely to become habit forming when used regularly.

Exercise Smart

Since exercise can have such a powerful effect on your blood glucose, it's important to be aware of the potential for hypoglycemia if you are on medications that increase this risk. For example, if your blood sugar were 100 mg/dL and you rode your bike for forty minutes, your blood glucose could drop to around 60 mg/dL, leading to uncomfortable, potentially dangerous symptoms. Since the effect of exercise lasts for hours, you could even develop a problem later that day.

Obviously we aren't trying to discourage you from exercising; we just want you to be smart about it. Here are some things to consider:

- When is the best time to exercise? Most people will find that it's after a light meal or snack.

- If you weren't planning to eat before exercising, check your blood glucose before you start. If it's less than 100 mg/dL, you may want to have a small snack first. Consider 15 to 30 grams of carbohydrate and a little protein. Some good examples include a six-ounce serving of yogurt, a piece of fruit and a serving of nuts, whole-grain crackers with peanut butter, or a hard-boiled egg with a slice of whole-wheat toast.

- Notice what happens six to twelve hours after exercise. Do a body-mind-heart scan and check your blood glucose. You may find that your glucose is lower all day.

Susan set a goal to walk for thirty to sixty minutes most days of the week. Here's what she discovered:

On Monday, I had my usual breakfast—whole-grain cereal with yogurt—and headed to the gym, where I walked on a treadmill for forty-five minutes. I felt great during exercise and for the rest of the day. Around four, I noticed that I was having trouble concentrating and felt hungry, so I checked my blood glucose. It was 88. This made me wonder what happens to my blood glucose on the days I exercise, so I decided to check it more frequently for a while. It's becoming clear that on the days I exercise, my blood glucose is more likely to be in the target range.

You're in charge of how active you are, so make time for your health and well-being. There are very few choices that you make each day that can have such a positive impact. If you're too busy for exercise, you're too busy. Write your own best prescription: what will you do, starting today, to move more and improve your health?

PART 3

Nonjudgment

Nothing is good or bad, but thinking makes it so.

—William Shakespeare

CHAPTER 9

Think:
What Do I Eat?

S o you're hungry. Good. Now you get to decide what to eat. At this point, we could give you a structured meal plan with a list of allowed foods and portion sizes to choose from, but that usually leads people back to a restrictive eating cycle, soon followed by an overeating cycle. Instead, think of Roger from chapter 1, a person who eats instinctively. What would he do?

He would eat what he wants. You might be thinking, *That's fine for him since he doesn't have diabetes, but I seem to want only "bad" food.* We have some good news for you. There are no "bad" foods. All foods can fit into a healthy diet, even when you have diabetes. That means *you* get to choose what you'll eat.

Erica has diabetes and is learning to use mindful eating to help her manage her blood glucose. Let's take a look at how she decides what to eat:

Yesterday was my birthday. My husband brought me breakfast in bed—scrambled eggs and toast—so I didn't take the time to check my blood sugar. They had planned a potluck at work for me too. It was going to be a good day!

I was hungry again by midmorning. I tend to get a little anxious about that, but I reminded myself that hunger is normal. I needed a snack but didn't want to eat too much because of the potluck, so I ate one of the oranges that I keep at my desk.

I checked my blood sugar before lunch and then looked over everything on the buffet table. I noticed that I was starting to feel uptight about all of the delicious things my coworkers had brought. I took a deep breath and did a quick body-mind-heart scan. I was at 2 on the hunger and fullness scale, so I filled half my plate with different veggies and salads and the rest with samples of other things that looked good to me. A couple of the dishes didn't live up to my expectations, so I just left them on my plate—and loved every bite of the ones that did!

In the middle of the afternoon, they surprised me with a birthday cake, candles and all. I was only at 4, but it was still yummy! About halfway through, I surprised myself by noticing that I was satisfied; I just left the rest on my plate.

Let's take a closer look at Erica's decisions. Erica typically eats breakfast every day (just not usually in bed!). She also makes a point of having healthy food available at her desk to eat when she gets hungry. She ate an orange to make sure she would be hungry again in time for the potluck. At lunch, Erica checked in. Although she initially felt a little anxious, she didn't try to avoid her favorites. Instead, she knew what her blood glucose was and how hungry she felt. She then served herself a balanced meal that was both healthy and delicious. Erica had cake for her afternoon snack. Although it wasn't her usual choice, she enjoyed every bite and stopped eating when she felt satisfied.

The most effective way to make permanent healthy lifestyle changes to manage your diabetes is to learn to eat according to your body's signals and to eat as healthfully as possible without feeling deprived. You can achieve this balance when you use reliable nutrition information to make your food choices while still allowing yourself the freedom to eat what you love without judging yourself or feeling guilty. Choosing food this way meets your natural need for nourishment and enjoyment.

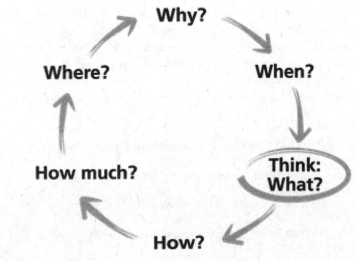

Figure 9.1

Erica's decision-making process can be summarized by three questions: *What do I want? What do I need? What do I have?* You can use these questions to help you make food choices that are healthful and satisfying and that support optimal glucose management.

What Do I Want?

Most of the time when you're hungry, a specific food, flavor, or texture comes to mind. As you get used to listening to your body's signals, you'll begin to recognize what type of food or taste matches your particular hunger at that time. Kim gave us a good example of why this is important:

> I was hungry and really wanted a few of the chocolate chip cookies I had bought for my kids' lunches. I've been trying to limit my carbs, so I ate a couple of slices of turkey instead. At first I felt good about it, but I just didn't feel completely satisfied. I decided to eat some baby carrots and then some cheese. Then I took a few bites from the ice cream carton, then a few more—for some reason, I always feel like I have to level off the top. I finally gave in and had the chocolate chip cookies after all. I felt so guilty that I ended up eating almost half the package before my kids came home. Afterward, I felt sick and thought, What did I accomplish here? It would have been better to eat two chocolate chip cookies in the first place and really enjoy them while I was actually hungry.

Satisfaction is not just physical fullness. Satisfaction comes from enjoying the food you eat. When you don't eat the food you really want, you may overeat other foods and eventually get around to eating what you wanted anyway. When you match the food you choose to what you're hungry for, you'll experience greater satisfaction and more enjoyment—with less food.

If a specific food doesn't come to mind, try to identify what you're hungry for by asking yourself these questions:

What taste do I want: sweet, salty, sour, spicy, or bitter?

What texture do I want: crunchy, creamy, smooth, or juicy?

What temperature do I want: hot, moderate, cold, or frozen?

What type of food do I want: light, heavy, or in between?

Do I want a certain category of food: protein, vegetables, or bread?

Is there a specific food I've been craving?

As you learn to ask yourself what you want, you'll discover that your body has wisdom. Listen to what Gary had to say:

When you said, "Ask yourself what you want," I was sure all I would eat was steak and potatoes—and I did, for a couple of days. Then I noticed I actually wanted a salad sometimes. By the end of the week, I was eating chicken, trout, fruit, soup, and even quiche. It was exciting to see what my taste buds would come up with next.

We've found that, like Gary, most people eventually gravitate toward balance, variety, and moderation when they begin asking themselves what they really want.

Eat What You Love

Let's face it. Food is wonderful. It's truly one of life's many pleasures. Enjoying food is only a problem if it's your *primary* source of pleasure.

The purpose of letting go of restrictive eating is to remove the false sense of value you place on certain foods. In essence, by letting go of guilt, you eliminate the power that certain foods have over you. Amazingly, your desire to overeat them usually diminishes.

The way to eliminate guilt is by giving yourself unconditional permission to eat *any* food. This means placing all foods on an even playing field, where the choice to eat cake evokes no more guilt than the choice to eat an apple. To eat without guilt, strive to:

- Stop judging foods as "good" or "bad."

- Eat what you really want, paying attention to your body's natural signals.

- Eat without having to pay penance (as in *I'll eat this today, but I'll be good the rest of the week* or *I'll eat this now, but I'll have to spend more time exercising tonight*).

Let Go of Fear-Based Thoughts

Even when you know that deprivation has led to overeating in the past, you may still be afraid to ask yourself what you're hungry for. If you've been stuck in an eat-repent-repeat cycle, you may doubt that you can freely choose to eat what you want without losing control. Remember: as you relearn to eat instinctively, you no longer have to be in control, just in charge.

Are you aware of any fear-based thoughts that can get in the way? Your beliefs and thoughts ultimately cause you to make certain decisions. By recognizing when your intention is being derailed by fear-based thinking, you can begin to think more fearless, empowering thoughts. Let's look at some examples:

Fear-based: I won't make healthy choices. You may be worried that if you ask yourself what you want, you'll always want sweets, fried food, or other foods you've tried to avoid. Initially, that may be true, especially if you've felt deprived.

Fearless: *I enjoy a variety of healthy, satisfying foods.* Once you let go of guilt about eating certain things, you'll gradually discover that you want a variety of foods to help you feel healthy and satisfied. Once you stop labeling foods as good or bad, you can develop a greater appreciation for the taste of fresh, healthful ingredients instead of seeing them as diet foods. In addition, you'll notice that you feel better physically and emotionally with a balance of nutritious foods, and your body will actually begin to crave them.

Fear-based: *I should feel guilty when I eat what I love.* Many popular food and diet ads feed into the fear that eating for pleasure is sinful and that you should eat only foods that are "guilt free."

Fearless: *I eat what I love, and I love what I eat.* In the long run, you'll be more satisfied if you choose a variety of foods you like, get rid of guilt, and make eating for enjoyment an intentional decision.

Fear-based: *I really shouldn't be eating this.* You are just giving yourself "pseudo permission" if you don't really believe you can eat certain foods. When you choose a food you think you shouldn't, instead of fully enjoying it, you'll plan to pay penance by exercising more, skipping your next snack or meal, or eating "light" to make up for it. Since you never really gave yourself permission to eat what you wanted, you will continue to feel out of control, overeat, and punish yourself for it: the eat-repent-repeat cycle.

Fearless: *I choose balance, variety, and moderation in my eating.* Give yourself unconditional permission to allow all foods in your diet. If you repeatedly overeat a particular food, notice what you are thinking and feeling. You may be in a subconscious restrictive eating cycle and setting yourself up for over-eating. All foods can fit into a balanced diet, so allow your common sense to guide your food choices by using the simple principles of balance, variety, and moderation.

Fear-based: *I'll use the hunger and fullness scale to control my eating.* Feeling guilty if you eat when you're not hungry or judging yourself for eating past level 5 or 6 is no different from dieting. This form of restrictive eating leads to the same eat-repent-repeat cycle.

Fearless: *I am in charge of all my decisions, including when I eat.* When you want to eat, ask yourself, *Am I hungry?*, knowing that you can choose to eat whether you are or not. Since being in charge means taking responsibility, you're free to choose to eat or overeat if you want as long as you acknowledge the possible consequences, such as discomfort or high blood glucose, and decide that for a given situation, the consequences are worth it.

Fear-based: I can't trust myself. You may believe you're addicted to certain foods, and you may feel afraid that you won't be able to stop eating them if you start. This is a self-fulfilling prophecy, because once you have even a bite, your mind automatically prepares for a binge. Depriving yourself of certain foods gives them power over you; in fact, it causes the strong cravings in the first place. This lack of self-trust comes from a history of cycling between overeating and restrictive eating.

Fearless: *I trust myself to eat in a way that nourishes my body, mind, and spirit.* When you know those previously forbidden foods will always be allowed, the urgency to eat them in large quantities eventually diminishes. People tire of eating the same kinds of food over time, even foods they love. Follow the steps outlined in "Strategies: Fearless Eating." Experiment with different foods and decide what foods you'll choose to eat based on how you respond.

Strategies: Fearless Eating

Are there foods that you'd love to be able to eat without guilt or fear? If so, the following strategies for fearless eating will help you rebuild trust in your ability to listen to your body wisdom. These steps will help you try out one previously forbidden food at a time and eat it regularly until it loses its magic and goes back to just being delicious. Move through the steps at a pace that's comfortable for you.

1. Make a list of your "scary foods," foods you enjoy but generally restrict yourself from eating for fear of losing control.

2. Choose one of the foods from your list and give yourself full permission to eat it when you're hungry and really, really, really, really want it. This is the "four really" test.

3. When you're hungry and decide you want that food (it passes the "four really" test), buy, prepare, or order one serving.

4. Eat the food mindfully, without distractions, and focus on the aroma, appearance, flavor, and texture as you eat. You'll learn more strategies for mindful eating in chapter 13.

5. Does the food taste the way you imagined it would? Sometimes you'll discover that it isn't as good as you thought it would be; you may even decide not to finish it or that you won't bother with it in the future. If you love it, continue to give yourself permission to buy or order it whenever you want.

6. You may decide to keep enough of that food in your house so that you'll know it's there if you want it. For some people, keeping certain foods in the house can feel too scary. In that case, promise yourself that you'll purchase and prepare only as much as you'll need for one sitting or go to a restaurant and order it when you want it.

7. Don't be surprised if you want that food frequently at first; that's normal. Relax; the cravings will decrease when you realize the food is no longer forbidden.

8. This strategy is also helpful if you find yourself obsessing about a particular food.

9. When you're ready, choose another food from your list and practice the process again.

10. If you find yourself overeating certain foods, ask yourself, *What was I thinking when I was eating it?* Thoughts like *I shouldn't eat this* or *I've already blown it; my sugar will be high anyway, so I might as well have another piece* can continue to drive overeating. Remember, you're in charge now, so replace those thoughts with more powerful, fearless thoughts.

11. Repeat these steps regularly to banish the fear that you're not in charge of your eating.

When you are free to eat whatever you want, you'll notice that food quickly loses the power and attraction it once had. You'll begin to trust that you can choose from among all the wonderful food choices available when you're hungry. You won't have to stock up in anticipation of your next round of self-denial. Amazingly, you'll also find that you make healthier choices and feel more satisfied with less food.

What Do I Need?

Food decisions are neither good nor bad, but clearly, some foods offer more nutritional benefits than others and affect your blood glucose in different ways. As you consider what food to choose, ask yourself, *What does my body need?*

Food fuels your body. It's wonderful to enjoy the food you choose, while keeping in mind that the main purpose of eating is to provide your body with the energy and nutrients it needs to function at its best. Since your body is the finest, most complex machine ever created, it performs best and lasts longest with top-of-the-line fuel. When you have diabetes, mindful eating helps you recognize how the type and amount of fuel affect the way this machine works.

So, how do you implement this in your daily life? Peter explains how he did it:

It felt great knowing that I'd never have to feel deprived again, but that didn't mean I wasn't interested in eating more healthfully. I decided to use my meter more regularly to see how carbs affect my blood sugar. As I learned more about carbohydrates, I wondered if I was eating enough fiber. I started reading food labels and realized that I was only eating around 15 grams of fiber a day, just half the 30 grams recommended. Now when I shop, I buy lots of vegetables, fruits, and beans. I look for high-fiber cereals, whole-wheat pasta, wild rice, and whole-grain bread. Within a few weeks, I was eating close to 30 grams of fiber a day. I feel better when I have fiber in my meals and snacks, and I notice that I feel fuller. Even my digestion is better.

Nourish Yourself

You can use food to your advantage when you learn to balance eating for nourishment with eating for enjoyment. Use the following strategies to help you with that process.

Make small, gradual changes. Forget all or nothing. Healthy eating is simply the result of all the little positive decisions you make.

Keep a blood glucose log. Monitoring your blood glucose consistently provides helpful feedback about your choices.

Choose food based on balance, variety, and moderation. Ask yourself what else you have been eating and what you are likely to eat later. Examples of helpful questions include *Have I eaten a variety of fruits and vegetables today? Have I been eating a lot of junk food or fast food lately? Do I eat too much protein or not enough? Do I feel tired when I eat too many carbohydrates in one meal? Have I been practicing balance, variety, and moderation over the last few days?* Your answers to questions like these will help you decide which foods you could choose to meet your nutritional needs.

Eat for overall health, not just diabetes management. They're not the same thing. If you only focus on eating low-carb foods without paying attention to the overall quality of your diet, your physical health and vitality will suffer.

Learn about nutrition. Use nutrition information to make informed decisions, not to deprive and punish yourself or to feel guilty. Pay close attention to the principles of balance, variety, and moderation. Surprisingly, once you know how one appealing food compares to another, you'll often find yourself preferring the more nutritious food.

The "Nourish" chapters provide information to help you understand the nutritional aspect of food. Without a doubt, science will continue to discover new and important information about nutrition and health. In fact, things are changing so rapidly in this field that even credible information from reliable sources may evolve and change over time. Find accurate and authoritative sources for nutrition information to keep up to date.

Be sure to examine how the information you learn applies to your life. Just because you hear or read something doesn't automatically mean you need to make a change. If you are unsure, your health care professional or a dietitian can help guide you through the maze of all the nutrition information that's available.

Consider your personal health needs. Take an honest inventory of your health. What specific issues do you need to consider when deciding what to eat? In addition to diabetes, think about the following issues and talk to your health care professional or a dietitian for specific recommendations if needed:

- Medical history (especially high cholesterol, high blood pressure, risk of cancer, kidney disease)

- Family history (especially high cholesterol, high blood pressure, cancer, heart disease)

- Allergies and reactions to certain foods (for instance, rashes, fatigue, digestive problems)

- Your health goals (for instance, target glucose, fitness, or weight loss)

Be willing to try new foods. You just might surprise yourself! It can take several tries of a new food to acquire a taste for it, but some of your favorite foods may turn out to be things you thought you wouldn't like. Don't persist in forcing yourself to eat foods you don't like, however, since that can backfire.

Make it taste great. Enjoy healthy choices by focusing on fresh foods, appealing combinations, new flavors, and interesting recipes. For example, learn to prepare healthy foods in exciting, delicious ways and learn to prepare your favorites in healthier ways by adjusting the ingredients or cooking method. Check out your local library or websites like www.diabetes.org for great recipes.

Look for healthful alternatives. Always ask yourself, *Is there a healthy choice that will meet my needs without leaving me feeling deprived?* For instance, could you decide to skip the fried appetizers and just enjoy the main course, order a great salad instead of a burger, or ask for a substitute for a less-healthy side dish with your favorite meal? The key is to make it a habit to choose more healthful foods unless you feel you really need to eat a particular food to feel satisfied.

Become aware of how you feel after you eat. Notice how long certain foods stay with you, whether you feel more energetic or sluggish after eating certain foods, and whether any foods cause uncomfortable symptoms. To put this in practical terms, here's what Bernice noticed:

I woke up late on Monday. I grabbed a cup of coffee with cream and sugar and headed out the door. On my way to work, I noticed I was hungry but realized I'd been in such a hurry that I had left my breakfast on the counter at home. I found a glazed doughnut when I got to work and settled for that. When I checked my blood sugar before lunch, it was high, so I didn't eat. I started to get hungry after my lunch hour. An hour later, I was shaky and foggy. When I checked my blood sugar, it was low, so I drank some juice and ate some candy. When I checked it again later, it was high.

On Tuesday, I woke up in time to have a cup of coffee and half a whole-wheat bagel with peanut butter. I didn't get hungry again for over three hours. My blood sugar was in the target range before lunch. I ate a turkey sandwich and a cup of vegetable soup for lunch, and I had almonds and grapes in the middle of the afternoon. I felt great all day.

By paying attention to the way her body responded to when, what, and how much she ate, Bernice was able to make different decisions that resulted in a more stable blood glucose, decreased hunger, and improved mood, attention, and performance. It's just one example of how mindfulness helps you feel your best and meet your nutrition needs.

Resist restrictive diets. Without a doubt, you'll continue to hear about many wonder diets that promise amazing results. You may even be tempted to try one. Before you do, carefully examine the premise and science behind it. A good rule of thumb is, if it sounds too good to be true, it is! Marilyn learned this the hard way:

I loved being in charge of my eating, and I was seeing slow but steady improvement in my hemoglobin A1c and the way I felt. But when my doctor told me my blood pressure was high, I decided to do something more drastic to lose weight. Everyone at work was buying diet shakes and supplements, so I spent about eighty bucks on a two-week supply. I lost four pounds the first week but gained it all back the second week. My blood sugar was crazy the whole time: up one minute, down the next. It took me weeks to get back on track again. Next time I decide to lose weight, I'll bump up my exercise, eat fewer sweets and more vegetables, and be sure that I'm using hunger and fullness to guide me.

Be open to more structure if needed. With diabetes, you have a medical reason for following a specific dietary plan. Having that structure can be really helpful—as long as you don't slip into restrictive eating. Even when you're following a meal plan, be sure to let hunger, satisfaction, and common sense guide you. A good rule of thumb here is this: if you can't imagine eating a certain way for the rest of your life, don't bother doing it for even a day. Eduardo knew he needed more structure:

I understood instinctive eating, but I was still having trouble stabilizing my blood sugar. I've never been able to stick with a diet for very long, but I knew I needed more support and accountability. My doctor referred me to diabetes classes, and I met with a dietitian who specializes in diabetes. We talked about what I like to eat and what changes I was ready to make, and then we agreed on a meal plan. I've been using the plan to help me choose what foods to eat, and I've been noticing my hunger and fullness signals to help me decide when to eat. She said it was just a guide and that I don't have to follow it perfectly to see improvement—and she was right. It doesn't feel anything like diets I've tried in the past.

When it comes to eating for health, being in charge means taking personal responsibility for your food choices. Combine your knowledge of nutrition with your personal lifestyle and preferences to choose food that works best for you, your diabetes, and your overall health.

What Do I Have?

This step can be summarized in one word: planning. Having a variety of foods available is critical if you're going to learn to use hunger to guide your eating. If you feel hungry and the only food available is from a vending machine, you'll probably choose a snack that may not be very healthy, may not taste very good, and may not really be what you were hungry for anyway.

Be prepared. The key is to keep a variety of foods available.

- Stock your home; workplace; and even your car, purse, or brief-case with different types of foods that meet the types of cravings you get. This way, you'll always have something satisfying available.

- Focus on healthful options that you enjoy when you're hungry but that won't be calling out to you, "I'm in here! Come eat me!"

- Ideas for low-carbohydrate options include precut vegetables, string cheese, nuts, hard-boiled eggs, light yogurt, cans of tuna, and slices of turkey or lean roast beef.

- Ideas for fiber-rich choices include packages of oatmeal, whole-grain crackers and breads, popcorn, whole-wheat pita chips, and fiber-rich snack foods.

- Buy or separate the food into appropriate portions. Small snack bags work great for this.

You're not always in charge of what's available, but you're still in charge of what and how much you choose. Remember to do your body-mind-heart scan first and then decide what you want and need before you survey your options for the best fit. Margo had a great way to be prepared at work:

I used to eat out for lunch nearly every day, mostly because it was conve-nient. I knew I was spending a lot of money and wasn't making the best choices for my health, so I decided to start taking my lunch to work. At the beginning of the week, I bring a small grocery bag full of lunch items like soup, lunch meat and whole-wheat bread, frozen dinners, crackers, yogurt, fruit, precut veggies, and even a few snack-sized candy bars. Now, no matter what I'm in the mood for, I can find something satisfying and am not as tempted to run out for a burger and fries.

If you're not used to choosing food mindfully and fearlessly, you may find it challenging at first. With practice, these strategies allow you to make choices that satisfy your body and mind. Eating food you truly enjoy while taking good care of your health is the best way to feel fully nourished.

CHAPTER 10

Care:
Taking Medication

The management of diabetes is like a three-legged stool: eating, physical activity, and, when needed, medications. When you use all three effectively, your blood glucose will likely be in an optimal range so that your diabetes will stabilize.

How Do You Feel about Taking Medication?

Pause for a moment to reflect on how you feel about taking medications, now or in the future. Let go of any judgment of yourself for your feelings; just notice.

It's normal to have strong feelings about taking medications. Some people feel guilty or ashamed because they feel they've failed at lifestyle management. Others are afraid because they believe that taking medications means their diabetes must be "really bad." Some are worried about side effects, risks, and the cost, as well as taking their medicines correctly. Some people are disappointed or frustrated because they don't like to take medication for any reason. Still others are relieved because they want to feel better and lessen their chances of having complications.

Whatever you experience, accept your feelings. They're not right or wrong, good or bad. They simply reflect your current beliefs about your situation. Resisting or shaming yourself for how you feel only creates stress that can sabotage your efforts to manage your blood glucose.

Why Do You Need Medication Anyway?

So far, this book has focused on lifestyle changes: why, when, what, how, and how much you eat, as well as where you invest your energy through physical activity and exercise. These are critical elements of mindful self-management. Why, then, are medications often necessary?

As you may recall from chapter 2, in type 1 diabetes, the pancreas is unable to produce insulin, which is why insulin must be taken immediately and for the rest of the person's life.

In type 2 diabetes, the onset is more gradual. The beta cells in the pancreas slowly lose the ability to make insulin due to insulin resistance caused by a genetic predisposition, age, diet, inactivity, weight gain, or some combination. Therefore, your eating and physical activity choices are two areas that you are in charge of for slowing down the progression from prediabetes to type 2 diabetes. As beta-cell function decreases, blood glucose rises, and medications become necessary for keeping your glucose in the target range. The Standards of Medical Care in Diabetes recommend starting metformin at the time of diagnosis of type 2 diabetes along with lifestyle changes to control glucose (ADA 2011).

You may wonder whether you will always have to take medications. Diabetes medications usually aren't stopped or changed unless there's a reaction to the medication or an intolerance of the side effects, or a medical reason to do so, such as a decrease in kidney function. It may help to remind yourself that the goal of diabetes self-management isn't to avoid medication but to keep your glucose in an optimal range for optimal health. When necessary, medications are used to achieve this goal. Remember, though, optimal management is a three-legged stool; medications don't replace diet and exercise. They all work together.

Why Are There So Many Medications?

You may wonder, *Why are there so many medications?*, or more important, *Why do I have to take so many pills or shots?* It's common for someone with diabetes to need more than one medication over time. There are many reasons—and none of them means you are a bad person!

Medications Work in Different Ways

Type 2 diabetes is actually a chain of events that occur in different parts of the body: the pancreas, liver, muscle, stomach, intestines, and cells. Therefore, medications have been developed that work on each of these different organ systems and their respective processes.

Medications Work at Different Rates

Some medications start working quickly, while others work more slowly. Some medications work for a short period, while others work all day. Therefore, you may need to take more than one medication if your blood glucose is elevated at different times during the day.

Medications Work Together

Medications often work synergistically. In other words, their total effect is greater than the sum of either one working alone. Your health care professional may combine medications to enhance their effectiveness, or more than one medication can be combined in a single pill.

Medications also have different side effects and risks, some of which only emerge at higher doses; instead of increasing the dose of a medication, a new one may be added.

Medications May Be Used Preventively

Some medications are used for prevention. For example, metformin may be prescribed for those at highest risk of developing diabetes (ADA 2011). ACE (angiotensin-converting enzyme) inhibitors or ARBs (angiotensin receptor blockers) may be prescribed to protect the kidneys from damage due to diabetes (Wolf and Ritz 2005), and low-dose aspirin may be recommended for people at increased risk of cardiovascular disease (Pignone et al. 2010).

Last, but not least, in addition to diabetes, insulin resistance often leads to high blood pressure and abnormal cholesterol profiles. These conditions are additional risk factors for heart disease. If lifestyle change has not been enough to control them, your health care professional will prescribe medications to treat these diseases too, which is essential to prevent complications.

Strategies: Mindful Medication Use

Since you are already familiar with the mindful eating cycle, let's ask the same questions for using medications more mindfully: why, when, what, how, how much, and where?

It's important to consult your health care provider and your pharmacist to be sure you have answers to any questions about your medications for maximal benefit and minimal side effects.

Why? Remember that your goal is to keep your glucose in an optimal range for optimal health. Be sure you understand why a particular medication is being used to help you achieve this goal. With that goal in mind, your awareness, your knowledge, and your glucose meter will all help monitor the effectiveness of your treatment. In addition, medications have different instructions, side effects, and risks. Have your health care professional, pharmacist, or diabetes educator write down specific directions and concerns when you start a new medication. Set up a follow-up phone call or appointment to review your blood glucose results, and discuss any symptoms or questions you have.

When? When you take the medicine and how often—the timing and frequency—are determined by how long it takes for the medication to start working, its peak onset of action, and how long it lasts in your system.

Find out if there is a specific time of day you should take the medication, for example, first thing in the morning or at bedtime.

If you take a medication more than once a day, be sure you understand when to take your doses. For example, are you supposed to take it before meals, in the morning and at bedtime, or on some other schedule?

Some medications are taken right before eating because they work quickly to control the rise of glucose levels. To prevent an episode of hypoglycemia, be sure to eat a meal that includes carbohydrate within ten to sixty minutes after taking this type of medication.

Some medications should be taken with meals, resulting in fewer side effects.

Pills or capsules that only need to be taken once a day often come in an extended-release formula that allows the medication to be released slowly. They usually can't be cut in half because that destroys the slow-release mechanism.

What? Be sure that each medication is clearly labeled with its name, dosage, instructions, and the reason you take it. Keep a complete list of all your medications (including over-the-counter medications, vitamins and supplements, and the type of glucose meter strips you use) with you at all times.

How? Some diabetes medications are taken as a pill, others as an injection. Taking your medications correctly and consistently improves their effectiveness.

How much? The required dosage of a medication is determined by its strength, the way it works in your body, and how your body responds to the medication. Don't try to compare the dose of one type of medication with that of another. That's like comparing apples to oranges.

Where? As described previously, knowing where your medication works in your body will help you understand more about using the medication properly and assessing its effectiveness.

What about Insulin?

If your body can no longer produce enough insulin to keep your blood glucose levels in the target range, then it's necessary to replace that insulin. For some people, this happens rapidly; for others, it's a more gradual process. Insulin cannot be taken orally because the digestive system would break it down. Therefore it must be "delivered," or injected, into the fat just below the skin, where it is absorbed into the bloodstream and sent to the rest of the body. Using insulin is not a last resort or a sign of failure. With appropriate education about its proper use, insulin is a safe and effective part of diabetes management."

Potential Weight Gain with Medication Use

Remember, in uncontrolled diabetes, glucose cannot get into your cells. Therefore, the level of glucose in your blood is high, and that glucose is eventually excreted in your urine. This process is very unhealthy and damages the organs, which is why diet, exercise, and medications are prescribed.

Again, remember to think of diabetes management as a three-legged stool. If medications alone are used to treat diabetes, weight gain can result when the calories that were previously trapped in the bloodstream and excreted in the urine are now available. Since weight gain can worsen insulin resistance, this can become a vicious cycle. Attention to your eating and physical activity will mitigate the side effect of weight gain, breaking the cycle.

You Are in Charge

Diabetes management is a dynamic process. There will be times when your blood glucose is easier to manage and times when it's more challenging, such as when you experience changes in your body and health, the aging process, stress levels, diet, and physical activity. Other changing circumstances include work, family, finances, travel, and other factors. Additionally, our understanding of diabetes continues to grow at a rapid pace. New research, new technologies, and new treatments make this an exciting field.

Admittedly, all of this can feel overwhelming at times. Remind yourself that change is normal and part of the process. By remaining in charge of your diabetes, you are committed to keeping your knowledge up to date and carefully choosing your health care team for its ability to provide the best treatment available. Choose to be mindful of how your treatment is working, and make sure that all three legs of your diabetes management stool support your goal of living healthy and well.

CHAPTER 11

Nourish:
Clearing Carbohydrate Confusion

C arbohydrates have gained a lot of attention recently, and sometimes what you hear is confusing, contradictory, or difficult to follow. Understanding the connection between the carbohydrates you eat and your blood glucose levels will help you take charge of your diabetes.

Why Are Carbohydrates Important?

As explained in chapter 2, the macronutrient carbohydrate provides your body with energy in the form of glucose. Plants manufacture all the carbohydrates found in foods, except for those in dairy products, which are made by cows that eat plants. Carbohydrates are found in bread and other grain products, legumes, starchy vegetables, fruit, dairy products, and sugar. Non-starchy vegetables also contain a small amount of carbohydrate.

Many carbohydrate-containing foods are also good sources of fiber and are nutrient rich; in other words, they are high in vitamins and minerals, such as B vitamins (thiamine, riboflavin, niacin), vitamin E, iron, zinc, calcium, selenium, and magnesium. A diet high in fruits, vegetables, whole grains, and fiber can reduce the risk of cardiovascular disease and cancer.

What Happens in Your Body?

At some point you may have heard someone say, "Carbs just turn to sugar in your body." Since sugar is another word for glucose, it's true that carbohydrate *does* turn into sugar during digestion. Since many people think of sugar as "bad," they also think of carbohydrates as "bad." Carbohydrates are not bad—even when you have diabetes. When you have diabetes, the shift is to become mindful of how much carbohydrate you eat at one time in order to manage your blood glucose level. To understand why, a brief science lesson is in order. (This may be a review for you, but since it's important, we'll try to make it as painless as possible.)

Insulin and Carbohydrates

When carbohydrates are eaten and digested, they're broken down to glucose molecules. Glucose then floats in your bloodstream (hence the term "blood glucose"), where it's ready to be used for energy or stored. While this explanation is oversimplified, under normal circumstances, the pancreas releases an appropriate amount of insulin to regulate the blood glucose level. (If you are still a little unclear about how all this happens, this is a good time to review chapter 2.)

With type 2 diabetes, your body resists the effects of insulin and is unable to produce enough insulin to maintain a normal glucose level. As a result, when you eat carbohydrate, your blood glucose level increases, but your body can't use the fuel efficiently, leading to symptoms like fatigue. In the long run, this extra glucose coats other tissues, eventually leading to the complications associated with diabetes.

Since carbohydrate-containing foods are an important source of fuel and nutrition for your body (and they are delicious!), understanding how to manage your glucose levels through eating, physical activity, and medications will help you make the best possible decisions for yourself. As you learned in chapter 9, when deciding what to eat, you can ask yourself three questions: *What do I want? What do I need? What do I have?* This chapter will focus on your decisions about carbohydrates.

Managing Your Carbohydrate Intake

Let's explore the two main factors that influence your glucose level when you eat carbohydrate-containing foods: the type of carbohydrate affects how fast the blood glucose rises, and the amount of carbohydrate affects how high it goes (Wheeler and Pi-Sunyer 2008).

Type of Carbohydrate

There are three main types of carbohydrate: sugar, starch, and fiber.

Sugar

Sugars are essentially small packages of glucose that your body breaks down easily and that raise your blood glucose quickly. Some foods are composed primarily of sugars; examples include table sugar, table syrup, corn syrup, honey, fruit juice, soda, and many types of hard candy.

Other sugars are found in combination with other nutrients: fructose in fruit and lactose in dairy products. Studies have shown that these carbohydrates seem to have less of an effect on blood glucose rise than other sugars (ibid).

Many people with diabetes mistakenly believe that sugar causes diabetes and that they aren't allowed to eat it. While sugar definitely raises blood glucose, it isn't necessary to eliminate it from your meal plan if you enjoy it. In fact, eliminating sugar isn't realistic and could lead to cravings, bingeing, and guilt. To take an old saying literally, then how can you "have your cake and eat it too"? In other words, how can you enjoy optimal blood glucose control while still including sweets in your meal plan if you want them? The keys, of course, are balance and moderation.

Starch

Starches are composed of long chains of glucose molecules. Although it takes longer for your body to digest starches than sugars, starch eventually breaks down into glucose and, therefore, causes your blood sugar to rise.

Foods that are high in starch include:

- Starchy vegetables, like peas, corn, potatoes, lima beans, and winter squash.

- Legumes, for example, dried beans, lentils, and peas, such as pinto beans, kidney beans, black-eyed peas, and split peas.

- Grains, like wheat, rice, oats, and barley, as well as grain products, such as bread, tortillas, pasta, cereal, and crackers. Whole grains and whole-grain products have important nutrients and fiber, whereas highly processed grains usually contain fewer nutrients and less fiber.

Non-starchy vegetables are low in carbohydrate—5 grams of carbohydrate or less per serving. Examples include salad greens, broccoli, cauliflower, cucumbers, and peppers.

Fiber

Dietary fiber, also known as roughage or bulk, includes the parts of plant foods that your body can't digest or absorb. A fiber-rich diet increases satiety, promotes smoother digestion, aids in preventing constipation, helps prevent certain diseases of the colon, and may reduce cholesterol levels. Several studies have also shown reduced risk of diabetes with increased intake of whole grains and dietary fiber (ADA 2008). The recommended fiber intake is approximately 25 grams per day for women and 38 grams per day for men, according to the USDA *Dietary Guidelines for Americans, 2010*. Most people eat only half of the recommended amount of fiber each day. Although it takes effort to meet the recommended fiber intake, the benefits are well worth it.

Here are a few tips for optimizing your fiber intake:

- When you choose bread, tortillas, crackers, pasta, rice, or cereal, look for whole-grain or whole-wheat varieties or ones that list brown rice or bran as the first ingredient. Check the food label for fiber content (the higher, the better). When foods have been highly processed or refined, the fiber content may be reduced or even eliminated.

- Look for high-fiber cereals; a pretty good guide is five or more grams of fiber per serving. If you aren't used to it, try mixing high-fiber cereal with your usual brand for a while.

- Use beans as a main course or add them to soups and salad for a filling meal. The soluble fiber found in beans, oats, oat bran, and flaxseed may help lower total blood cholesterol levels.

- Eat apples, potatoes, and other fruits and vegetables with their skins when possible, since there's a lot of fiber in the skin.

- Fruits with seeds, like raspberries and blackberries, are also higher in fiber.

- Eat whole fruits instead of drinking juice.

Joseph shared what he noticed:

I had always heard that a high-fiber diet was healthier, so I made whole-wheat pasta and added veggies like peppers, squash, and mushrooms, and I served myself a large salad—nearly three cups! I can usually eat a lot of pasta, but with all the vegetables and salad, I found I got fuller faster and I couldn't eat all the food on my plate. As a result, I noticed that my blood glucose was lower than usual. Even more interesting was that I didn't get hungry after dinner so I didn't snack that night! I'm going to experiment with other high-fiber foods now too.

Amount of Carbohydrate

The USDA Dietary Guidelines for Americans, 2010 recommends that 45 to 65 percent of your total calorie intake come from carbohydrate. However, having diabetes requires a shift from thinking about your daily total to the amount of carbohydrate you eat at each meal or snack. To help you do this, we describe two meal planning techniques below: planning your plate using carbohydrate choices and counting carbohydrates.

The purpose is to help you keep your carbohydrate intake at a level that won't exceed your body's ability to process the glucose. It also gives you the flexibility to select foods at each meal or snack that will be most satisfying to you at that time, while keeping your blood glucose levels in target. (Can you see how checking your blood glucose will provide you with feedback about how much carbohydrate your body can handle?)

The recommended dietary allowance for digestible carbohydrate is a minimum of 130 grams, though you may need more to meet your energy needs. A dietitian or a certified diabetes educator can help you learn how to plan meals and how many carbohydrates to eat at each meal. Generally, having 45 to 60 grams of carbohydrate per meal is a good place to start. As you learned in chapter 6, using your blood glucose log to make notes about your hunger and fullness levels, carbohydrate intake, blood glucose levels, and physical activity will help you work with your health care team to determine the right amount of carbohydrate for you.

Planning Your Plate Using Carbohydrate Choices

Using the method introduced in chapter 7, start by filling half your plate with low-carbohydrate vegetables, which are typically nutrient and fiber rich and relatively low in carbohydrate and calories (see the following table of Low-Carbohydrate Vegetables for examples). You'll also select a source of protein; you'll learn more about that in chapter 19.

Low-Carbohydrate Vegetables

Each serving below contains less than 5 grams of carbohydrate

Typical Serving Sizes

Salad greens .... 2 cups

Raw .... 1 cup

Cooked .... 1/2 cup

Examples: beets, broccoli, carrots, cauliflower, celery, cucumbers, eggplant, green beans, green-leafy vegetables (beet greens, collard greens, kale, lettuce, spinach, Swiss chard), mushrooms, okra, onions, parsnips, peppers, squash (spaghetti, summer, zucchini), turnips

Figure 11.1

The carbohydrate-containing foods that have the greatest effect on your blood glucose are located in the upper-right portion of the Eat What You Love with Diabetes illustration (Figure 7.1): grains, starchy vegetables, dairy, and fruit. The following table, Carbohydrate Choices, lists examples of *carbohydrate choices* containing approximately 15 grams of carbohydrate per serving. For example, a woman who eats 45 to 60 grams of carbohydrate at each meal would select three to four carbohydrate choices. A man who eats 60 to 75 grams of carbohydrate per meal would select four to five carbohydrate choices. If you want to include a dessert with your meal, you can replace one or more of your other carbohydrate choices with the desired sweet.

Carbohydrate Choices

Each serving below contains approximately
15 grams of carbohydrate

Grains and Grain Products

Bread*..1 slice

Cereal (cold)*..2/3 cup

Cereal (hot)*...1/2 cup

Crackers*...6

Hamburger bun, English muffin 1/2

Popcorn... 3 cups

Rice, pasta ....1/3 cup

Beans and Starchy Vegetables

Beans (black, chickpeas, lentils, pinto) ....1/2 cup

Potato, baked or boiled...1/2 medium

Potato, mashed ....1/2 cup

Peas, corn ....1/2 cup

Winter squash... 1 cup

Fruit

Berries..3/4–1 cup

Canned fruit in its own juice*.............................. 1/2 cup

Cherries, grapes 12–15

Fresh fruit .... 1 small

Fresh fruit, cut up .... 1 cup

Fruit juice..1/2 cup (4 ounces)

Dairy

Milk... 1 cup

Yogurt, plain or light*.............................3/4 cup (or 6 ounces)

Sweets

Ice cream* ....1/2 cup (4 ounces)

Regular soda* .... 4 ounces

Sandwich cookies*.. 2 small (1 ounce)

Sugar or honey*.. 1 tablespoon

Vanilla wafers*.. 5 wafers (1 ounce)

*Check the label

Figure 11.2

If you're hungry between meals, you may decide to include one or two carbohydrate choices (15 to 30 grams of carbohydrate) in a snack.

Paul shares how learning to use carbohydrate choices helped him:

At first, I thought I was only allowed to eat half a potato or half an English muffin. It seemed so silly to me; what are you supposed to do with the other half? Now that I understand that a carbohydrate choice is the amount of food equal to 15 grams of carbohydrate, it's easy to see that the foods that are higher in carbohydrates have smaller portion sizes. I also understand that it doesn't mean that's all I'm allowed to eat! It just means I can easily keep track of the carbohydrates based on how many choices I actually eat.

Carbohydrate Counting

Another way to manage your carbohydrate intake is to keep track of the number of carbohydrates you eat throughout the day. You can even download applications for your mobile phone that make it easier to do this. Figure out how much carbohydrate the foods you eat have by checking the food label or looking it up online. Many restaurant chains also have nutrition information (including carbohydrate content) on their websites, and some fast-food restaurants have nutrition pamphlets available onsite.

Be sure to look at the serving size first since the rest of the information is based on this portion. Next, find the "Total Carbohydrate." Look for the first number, which is followed by a "g" for grams. This is the total amount of carbohydrate in one serving of that food, including starches, sugars, and fiber. If you eat more or less than one serving, you need to do a little math to figure out the amount of carbohydrate you consumed. With a little practice using these techniques, you'll see which method works best for you. Susan likes to think in terms of slices of bread:

If I look at a food label or list and see that a food has 15 grams of carbohydrates per serving, I think of this as equal to a slice of bread. If it has 30 grams, it's equal to two slices of bread, and so on. I was really surprised to learn that the bagel I was getting from my favorite coffee shop had 78 grams of carbohydrates. I was basically eating five slices of toast for breakfast! No wonder my blood sugar was high.

You Eat Food, Not Just Carbohydrates

To restate an important point from chapter 7, you don't consume nutrients; you eat food. For people who love to eat, this is a very good thing! Naturally, it also means that there is interplay between the foods you eat and their effect on your blood glucose and satiety. Variables like cooking method and time, amount of heat or moisture used, ripeness of fruits and vegetables, and degree of processing affect the blood glucose response. In addition, most foods contain a mixture of macronutrients (carbohydrate, fat, and/or protein) and many meals and snacks are a combination of different foods—cheese and crackers, meat and potatoes, stir-fried chicken and vegetables over rice—to name just a few of the thousands of options.

Through your awareness of hunger and fullness, you may discover that protein-containing foods lead to the greatest level of satiety, followed by fat and then carbohydrates. If this is true for you, you can experiment with your snacks and meals to manage your blood glucose levels and match your preferred eating style, medication schedule, and physical activity patterns. By managing your carbohydrate intake and experimenting with adding protein, healthy fats, and fiber to your snacks and meals, you can stabilize your blood glucose and hunger levels.

Taryn's curiosity helped her understand how the type and amount of carbohydrate, along with the other macronutrients she ate at the same time, influenced her blood glucose, energy, and hunger levels:

> I have a sweet tooth. Finding out I had diabetes didn't make it go away. I quickly discovered that eating too much candy, cake, or cookies caused my blood sugar to spike, my energy level to drop, and my hunger to come back a short time later. I began experimenting a little. Now, when I'm hungry and in the mood for sweets, I'll have something like two cookies with a cup of skim milk. If I plan to have dessert after dinner, I eat fewer carbs during my meal and make sure I'm not too full to enjoy dessert. My blood sugars don't spike the way they used to, and I like that I get to decide what I'll eat.

Here again, mindful eating and a sense of curiosity are helpful for noticing patterns and choosing what you'll eat from one meal to the next. We'll continue to explore this concept further in the remaining "Nourish" chapters. Before long, you'll be an expert at understanding your body's signals.

Healthy Eating Tips

Here are practical tips for healthier eating:

- Eat plants. Plant foods are packed with nutrients and help fill you up and boost your fiber intake. Look for whole grains and whole-grain products. Go for fruits and vegetables with deeply colored flesh, such as mangoes, blueberries, cantaloupe, tomatoes, red peppers, and dark leafy greens, since they generally have more micronutrients. Eat edible skins and peels (thoroughly washed) to increase your fiber and nutrient intake.

- Give yourself plenty of time for grocery shopping; it's challenging to learn more about your options when you're rushed. Make a list before you go to the store. This helps you think about what you need so that you don't fall into old habits and respond to external food cues. Shop the perimeter of the grocery, where all the most nutritious foods are, only venturing up the aisle for items on your list.

- Pick one type of food and learn more about the choices available. For example, if you compared three or four different types and brands of tomato sauce, you might learn that some have two grams of carbohydrates, while another has 15 grams. Pick a different food product to learn about each time you go to the store.

- For variety, try one of the many exciting and flavorful grains. Look for wild rice, basmati rice, jasmine rice, barley, bulgur, couscous, quinoa, polenta, and kasha. Cook according to package directions, or use vegetable or chicken broth in place of water. Add fresh or dried herbs, a small amount of olive oil, flavored vinegar, and diced vegetables for a hot side dish or cold salad.

- Add vegetables and beans to your stews, soups, rice, pasta, or frozen entrées to boost the nutrients and fiber content. Some examples are spinach in meat loaf, shredded carrots in spaghetti sauce, kidney beans in chili, and chopped broccoli in rice pilaf.

- Make flavorful grilled vegetables. Just marinate asparagus, sliced peppers, eggplant, portobello mushrooms, zucchini, or onions in a dressing, or brush them with olive oil and sprinkle with seasoning and grill or broil. Serve as a gourmet side dish or snack, and use the leftovers in sandwiches, salads, pizzas, and pastas.

- Aim for three servings a day of dairy. Dairy products are nutrient rich, containing protein; calcium; vitamins A, D, B$_{12}$, and riboflavin; phosphorus; and magnesium.

- Keep ready-to-eat fruits on hand—fresh, whole fruits or dried fruit—as a convenient, sweet, high-fiber snack that often satisfies a sweet tooth.

- You might also be interested in experimenting with nonnutritive sweeteners to add sweetness without overdoing it. Keep in mind that just because something is "sugar free" doesn't mean that it's carbohydrate free, fat free, or healthful. Awareness and moderation are the best rules of thumb.

Eating for Overall Health

Although managing your carbohydrate intake helps you manage your blood glucose, it's important to keep the big picture in mind: eating for overall health and enjoyment. And while it's easy to become distracted by all the numbers, remember to decide how hungry you are before you eat and notice how full you are afterward. With practice, you'll discover that your body will guide you to eat the amount of food it needs.

CHAPTER 12

Live:
Increase Your Stamina

Perhaps you're already convinced of the benefits of exercise for good health and well-being. Let's focus on the ways specific types of exercise will help you, beginning with building your stamina through cardiorespiratory fitness.

Simply put, cardiorespiratory (*cardio* means "heart," and *respiratory* means "breathing") exercise, commonly called "cardio," is any activity that increases your heart rate and breathing. As a result, it strengthens your heart, lungs, and vascular system, and it improves circulation throughout your body.

Why Bother?

Cardiorespiratory activity offers numerous health benefits (ACSM and ADA 2010). Some are directly related to your blood glucose management, while others reduce your risk of cardiovascular disease and improve your overall health and well-being. Cardiorespiratory activity:

- Lowers your blood glucose

- Reduces insulin resistance

- Prevents or delays the onset of type 2 diabetes

- Reduces the amount of medication needed to manage your blood glucose

- Conditions your heart, lungs, and vascular system

- Lowers your blood pressure and resting pulse

- Raises your level of HDL cholesterol, the "good" cholesterol

- Lowers your risk of developing cardiovascular diseases such as heart attack, stroke, and atherosclerosis (hardening of the arteries)

- Increases your stamina

- Helps you lose excess body fat

- Strengthens your major muscles and creates a more toned appearance

- Improves your sense of well-being

- Improves your sleep

- Boosts your energy level

What You Need to Know

There are many cardiorespiratory activities to choose from, including walking, cycling, water aerobics, swimming, dancing, low-impact aerobics, hiking, jogging, skating, stair stepping, tennis, rowing, cross-country skiing, jumping rope, basketball, soccer, and more. Even gardening and housework can be a good workout. As you can see, the list includes a variety of activities for all fitness levels, so there's something for everyone.

No matter which activity you choose, the goal is to keep your heart rate up without completely losing your breath. Since each person is at a different fitness level, an activity that's comfortable for one person may be too much for someone else. For example, jogging might be a perfect activity for someone who exercises regularly, while a person who's just getting started might feel totally winded within a short period and have to quit. The person who is just starting out will benefit far more from walking and will get just as good a workout for his or her current level of fitness. The point is, start wherever you are.

Getting Started

Walking is an ideal activity for almost any fitness level, because you can walk just about anywhere, anytime, with minimal equipment. Before you take your first step, make sure you're prepared to enjoy it.

Exercise smart. Be sure to get clearance from your health care professional before starting any exercise program. Review chapter 8 for tips on exercising safely with diabetes and preventing problems with hypoglycemia.

Care for your feet. When you have diabetes, your feet need special care. Be sure to check your feet before and after exercise for any unusual swelling, redness, pain, sores, cuts, or blisters. Seek medical care immediately for any of these signs or symptoms. Wear comfortable shoes with flexible, thick soles, preferably shoes that have been designed for walking. Check your shoes before wearing them to make sure there's nothing inside the shoe that could irritate or injure your feet. Wear socks that fit correctly to decrease friction and prevent blisters.

Wear appropriate clothing. Comfortable, light cotton clothing absorbs sweat and allows evaporation in summer. Wear layers of clothes in winter because you'll quickly warm up with activity. Don't be too concerned with how you look: the goal is to feel good.

Choose a location. Your neighborhood is the best place to start, if possible, since it's the most convenient. Having a treadmill at home also makes it convenient to walk anytime. For variety and interest, walk in nearby neighborhoods, parks, and malls or on walking trails. Look for smooth, even surfaces if you are not very sure footed. Surfaces softer than concrete may be more comfortable. Try a track at the local high school, or walk on the asphalt rather than the sidewalk, being very mindful of traffic, of course.

Consider safety. In addition to carrying glucose tablets with you and wearing a medical identification bracelet if you are at risk for hypoglycemia, take precautions for your general safety. Walk in the daytime or in well-lit areas. Wear reflective clothing or shoes if you walk at night. Stay aware of your surroundings. Let others know your route and expected time of return, and take your cell phone with you if possible. Consider carrying pepper spray and a whistle or another type of alarm to use in case you encounter danger. Walking with a partner provides additional security.

Use sun protection. Don't forget to wear a hat, sunscreen, and sunglasses with UVA and UVB protection during the peak hours of the day—even during the winter.

Use proper walking technique. Walk with your head and chin up, shoulders held slightly back, and stomach pulled in. Touch your heel to the ground first and then roll your weight forward. Make sure your toes point straight ahead. Swing your arms as you walk, either down at your side or with your elbows flexed to 90 degrees, with your fist swinging up to the level of your breastbone.

Take a partner. If you like the idea of sharing your walk with someone else, choose one or more partners who can walk on the same schedule and who are at about the same level of fitness or higher. This is a great chance to spend quality time with someone, and it definitely keeps you motivated and makes the time go faster. Pets or children on bikes or in strollers make good partners too.

One Step at a Time

Many people choose walking as their cardiorespiratory activity, so we'll use that as our example. If walking is not a good activity for you, choose something else you might enjoy. No matter what you choose to do, start slowly, be consistent, and keep it interesting.

The American College of Sports Medicine (ACSM) and the American Diabetes Association (ADA 2011) recommend exercising for a total of 150 minutes a week (that is an average of 30 minutes, five days a week). They suggest that you not go more than two days between bouts of activity because the beneficial effects wear off. If you are just getting started, use the following chart to work your way up to 30 minutes. You can also break your walk into several shorter sessions if you're too busy or not used to exercising; you'll still get the benefits.

The "best" time to exercise is whenever you'll do it most consistently. Many people find it easier to be consistent when they exercise in the morning after a light breakfast, before other distractions get in the way. Of course, the bonus is increased energy and less stress throughout the rest of the day.

At the beginning of the week, schedule your walks and write them down on your calendar. Once you've committed yourself to those times, give them the priority they deserve. If you have to cancel, reschedule just as you would any other important appointment.

The following sample schedule is one way to build your cardiorespiratory fitness with walking. If you haven't been exercising regularly, start at the top and gradually work your way from fifteen minutes up to sixty. If you're already exercising, simply choose the starting point that matches your current fitness level, and go from there. This is just a sample, so make adjustments to meet your needs. You can also use this sample chart to build activities other than walking.

Sample Walking Schedule

Week	Warm-Up	Brisk Walk	Cool Down	Total Time	Stretching
1	5 min	5 min	5 min	15 min	After walk
2	5 min	7 min	5 min	17 min	After walk
3	5 min	10 min	5 min	20 min	After walk
4	5 min	12 min	5 min	22 min	After walk
5	5 min	15 min	5 min	25 min	After walk
6	5 min	18 min	5 min	28 min	After walk
7	5 min	21 min	5 min	31 min	After walk
8	5 min	24 min	5 min	34 min	After walk
9	5 min	27 min	5 min	37 min	After walk
10	5 min	30 min	5 min	40 min	After walk

Each walking session should be made up of four parts:

Warm up: Walk slowly for five minutes and allow your muscles to warm up by increasing your circulation. Please note that warming up is not the same thing as stretching. Stretching is best after the muscles are warm, usually after your warm-up and at the end of your walk.

Brisk walk: Gradually increase your intensity as you begin to feel more energetic. You should be able to carry on a conversation, but if you can sing, go a little faster. As you become more fit, increase your intensity and time by walking a little faster and adding a few extra minutes to challenge yourself.

Cool down: Walk slowly for five minutes to allow your muscles to cool down and your circulation to return to normal.

Stretch: Stretching after your warm-up and again at the end of your walk will help prevent injuries. (Chapter 24 provides the details to get you started.)

Walking is a fun and very effective way to get fit and increase your energy, reduce insulin resistance, improve your blood glucose levels, and decrease your risk of heart disease. By adjusting the frequency (how often), intensity (how much effort you use), duration (how long you walk), and type (alternating walking with other cardiorespiratory activities, like hiking, swimming, dancing, or bike riding), you can create a program that's just right for you.

Fitness Rx: FITT Formula for More Stamina

The FITT Formula—frequency, intensity, time, and type—can be used to help you build more stamina.

- *Frequency:* Exercise most days of the week.

- *Intensity:* Use enough effort to challenge yourself.

- *Time:* Aim for anywhere from ten to sixty minutes, continuously or broken up into shorter sessions.

- *Type:* Do any activity that elevates your heart rate and makes you breathe harder.

Keep It Interesting

- Don't get stuck in a rut. Try a longer session once in a while, a different time of day, a new path, or a walking partner. Vary your walking environment; try walking on a treadmill, outdoors on pavement, through a wooded trail, up and down hills, even in water.

- A pedometer is a fun way to measure your activity level throughout the day, both during routine activities and while exercising. It measures the number of steps you take or the distance you walk, making it easy to set small goals for yourself. It's really motivating to see those steps add up—and to see your energy level rise as your fitness improves.

- Continually challenge yourself so that your fitness level continues to improve. You can increase how long, how far, or how frequently you walk. Increase the intensity of your walk by going faster, moving your arms, pushing a stroller, walking uphill, jogging for short periods, or using the fitness programs on your treadmill.

- Try new cardiorespiratory activities. This keeps you from getting bored and uses different muscle groups to improve your overall fitness. Try activities like swimming, cycling, hiking, dancing, jogging, rowing, cross-country skiing, tennis, exercise classes, exercise tapes, and others.

- Sign up to participate in a charity walk or run. It's a fun way to raise money and increase awareness for your favorite causes while adding a little motivation.

- Try meditative walking to clear your mind while you are exercising your body. For example, inhale slowly for four steps, hold your breath for one step, exhale slowly for four steps, and then hold for one step. Repeat.

Building your cardiorespiratory fitness has many benefits for your blood glucose, health, weight, stamina, and energy. Choose activities you think you'll enjoy, create a plan, and keep it interesting. By taking it one step at a time, you'll find yourself on your way to optimal health.

PART 4

Being Present

[T]he meeting of two eternities, the past and future…
is precisely the present moment.

—Henry David Thoreau, *Walden*

CHAPTER 13

Think:
How Do I Eat?

You're now more aware of the decisions you need to make about why, when, and what you eat. Now decide how you'll eat.

Ironically, people often say they love food, but they don't eat in a way that shows this. For example, do you eat quickly, barely tasting what you're eating? Do you eat too fast to notice how full you're getting? Do you eat while watching TV, reading the newspaper, driving, or working? How often do you feel stuffed after eating? Do you ever finish something and wish for just one more bite? Have you ever eaten something and not even remembered it?

These are all signs of mindless or unconscious eating. Your brain and body cannot process information fully when you eat too quickly or when you're distracted by something else (Oldham-Cooper et al. 2011).

On the other hand, think about one of your most memorable eating experiences. If you were writing an article about your meal for a gourmet magazine, how would you describe the location, your companions, your conversation, the ambience, the appearance and aroma of the food, its taste, and your feelings while eating and afterward?

How often do you have eating experiences like that? How often would you like to have experiences like that? Mindfulness changes eating into a memorable, multisensory experience.

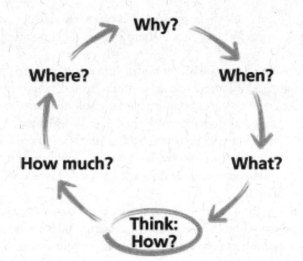

Figure 13.1

Love What You Eat

Eating is a natural, healthy, and pleasurable activity for meeting your body's needs. Choosing to eat mindfully—that is, eating with *intention* and *attention*—will give you optimal enjoyment and satisfaction from eating.

Eat with *intention*. Be purposeful when you eat.

- Eat when you're truly hungry.

- Eat to meet your body's needs.

- Eat with the goal of feeling *better* when you're finished.

Eat with *attention*. Devote your full attention to eating.

- Eliminate or minimize distractions.

- Tune in to the ambience, flavors, smells, temperature, and texture of the food.

- Listen to your body's cues of hunger and fullness.

When you eat with the intention of caring for yourself, you'll feel contented, not deprived. When you pay attention, you'll enjoy eating more while eating less.

Mindful eating helps you recognize the difference between physical satisfaction and fullness. When you eat on autopilot, you may only become aware when you're overly full. But at comfortable satiety, level 5 or 6 on the Hunger and Fullness Scale, your stomach may be just slightly distended. At that point, you could eat more, but your body isn't asking for it. Because it's a very subtle feeling of stomach fullness (less obvious than the signal to start eating), you must listen to your body carefully or you'll miss it. This is one place where mindfulness comes in.

Another benefit of mindful eating is that you'll notice how you feel, both physically and emotionally, when you eat certain foods, eat in certain environments, or eat in certain ways. This may affect your future choices about eating.

It's important to observe how you eat from a neutral perspective. In other words, don't judge or punish yourself for the way you eat. Instead, use your heightened awareness to increase your satisfaction from eating. Here's how Rhonda explained it:

> I always said I couldn't control my diabetes because I love food too much. As I learned more about mindful eating, I realized I needed to love eating more, not less. I ate dinner while I watched television or read a book, so I could barely remember what I ate, much less how it tasted. I'd finish off a bag of chips without even noticing. When I'd eat something delicious, it was hard to stop. Afterward, I'd realize that it had stopped tasting good long before I had stopped eating. I'd feel miserable, and, of course, my blood sugar would be high.
>
> Mindful eating has opened a world of possibilities. I don't eat out of habit anymore. I try new foods and new recipes because I love the experience. I don't eat as much, but I love it more!

You can experience eating with intention and attention by practicing these steps for mindful eating, either by yourself or with a friend over dinner. Use the mindful eating cycle as your guide. If you have not learned the steps in the cycle already, this would be a good time to commit them to memory (review figure 1.1). That way you can easily recall them as you practice.

Why?

Acknowledge why you're eating. Are you eating for fuel, nutrition, pleasure, convenience, or because of a physical, environmental, or emotional trigger? Why you're eating will affect every other decision in your eating cycle. Notice how certain situations, social occasions, and emotions affect what, how, and how much you eat. When you're aware of why you're eating, you're more in charge of the rest of the decisions you make.

When?

Become present. Get in the habit of checking in with yourself several times a day to see where you are on the Hunger and Fullness Scale. Begin eating when you feel significantly hungry (level 2 or 3), but try not to wait until you're famished (level 1). One of the keys to mindful eating is to keep your body adequately fed to decrease the risk of overeating.

Set your intention. Decide how full you want to be after eating. Aim for a specific number on the Hunger and Fullness Scale. Remember, you're in charge of how much you eat, but if you don't have a plan, you're more likely to eat more than you want or need.

What?

Choose food that will satisfy both your body and mind. To get the optimal level of satisfaction from your food, remember to ask yourself these three questions: *What do I want?*, *What do I need?*, and *What do I have?* Review chapter 5, if necessary.

How?

Purchase, prepare, or serve only the amount of food you think you'll need. With practice, you'll be able to predict how much food it will take to fill you up at different levels of hunger. If someone else filled your plate, visually determine how much you think you'll need, and move or remove the excess. If you're at a restaurant, ask for a to-go container before you start eating.

Create a speed bump. Once you have the amount of food you think you'll need, physically divide it in half on your plate to remind yourself to stop halfway and check in again. This little "speed bump" will slow you down and serve as a reminder to become mindful again if you've lost your focus. When you reach that point, you'll stop eating for two full minutes to reconnect with your hunger and fullness level.

Create a pleasant environment. A pleasant ambience adds to your enjoyment and satisfaction from eating. Even when you're preparing food for yourself, make it attractive, as if you were serving it to someone special (you are!). Set the table, turn on music, and maybe even light candles. Even a frozen dinner looks more appealing on a nice plate.

Minimize distractions. If you eat while distracted by television, reading, driving, working, or talking on the telephone, you won't be able to give your food or your body's signals your full attention. Consequently, you may feel full but not satisfied. Some people say they get bored when they "just eat." That's particularly true as your hunger begins to fade, so use boredom as a signal that it's time to stop.

Calm yourself. If you're upset, anxious, or excited, take some time to calm down before you begin eating. Likewise, avoid having stressful conversations at the dinner table.

Sit down. Eating while standing over the sink, peering into the refrigerator, or propped up in bed makes it difficult to stay aware. Instead, choose one or two areas at home and at work for eating. This also breaks or prevents the formation of triggers associated with other locations.

Center yourself. Take a few deep breaths to calm and center yourself before you begin eating. This will help you slow down and give eating your full attention.

Express gratitude. In your way, take a moment to reflect on and give thanks for your food and the nourishment it provides. Appreciate the earth, air, and water for their contributions to your meal. Think for a moment of all the people who invested their time, effort, and talent to get the food to your plate.

Look at your food. Appreciate the appearance and aroma. Notice the colors, textures, arrangement, and smells. Imagine what it will taste like.

Taste your favorite first. Decide which food looks the most appetizing and start by eating one or two bites of it while your taste buds are the most sensitive. If you save the best until last, you may want to eat it even if you're full—and you won't enjoy it as much.

Put your fork down. When you're loading your next forkful, you can't pay attention to the one in your mouth. Besides, when you're always paying attention to the next bite, you'll keep eating until there are no more bites because that's where your focus is.

Stay connected. Savor the aromas and tastes of your food as you eat. Mentally describe the temperatures, flavors, ingredients, seasonings, and textures. Stay conscious of all the different sensations you're experiencing.

Take small bites. Large bites are wasted on the roof of your mouth, teeth, and cheeks, where you have very few taste buds. In addition, much of the flavor of food comes from the aromas. When you slowly chew a small bite of food, the aromas are carried from the back of your throat to your nose, enhancing the taste.

Appreciate the occasion. Appreciate the atmosphere, the company, or simply the fact that you're allowing yourself to sit down and enjoy your meal.

Enjoy the food. If you notice you're not enjoying what you chose, choose something else if possible. Eating food that doesn't taste good to you will leave you feeling dissatisfied.

How Much?

Pause in the middle of eating. When you get to your speed bump, take a break from eating for at least two full minutes. Ask yourself where you are on the Hunger and Fullness Scale now. Estimate how much more food it will take to fill you to comfortable satiety, keeping in mind that there's a delay in the fullness signal reaching the brain. Don't be surprised if you realize you're already full or getting close.

Notice when your taste buds become less sensitive to the taste of food. When the food doesn't taste as good as it did at first, it's a sign that your body has had enough.

Push your plate forward or get up from the table as soon as you feel satisfied. The desire to keep eating will pass quickly, so direct your attention away from food for a few minutes. Remind yourself that you'll eat again when you're hungry again.

Notice where you are on the Hunger and Fullness Scale after eating. How close did you get to your original intention?

Where?

Notice where your fuel is after eating. How do you feel? If you overate, don't judge or punish yourself. Just notice the physical or emotional discomfort, or both, that often accompanies being overly full, and create a plan to decrease your likelihood of overeating next time. (We'll address this in more detail in the next chapter.)

Where will you invest the energy you consumed? Remember that the purpose of eating is to fuel living. Where will your energy go? (You'll find more on this in chapter 21.)

Strategies: Eating Mindfully in the Real World

It's easier to become distracted from noticing signals of physical hunger and satiety at restaurants and social gatherings, especially when food is the main event. Eating mindfully in the workplace also poses some common challenges. In these environments, you may need to pay extra attention to your body's signals.

- Remember to ask yourself, *Am I hungry?* It's common to see dishes of candy or snacks at parties and in many places of business, but don't eat food just because it's there. Before having a doughnut, bagel, or brownie from the break room at work or a sample at the grocery store, notice where you are on the Hunger and Fullness Scale. If you're hungry and really want that food, remember to sit down and eat it mindfully. If you're not hungry, save some of it for later or skip it altogether. It will probably reappear another day.

- Be mindful about eating at your desk. Make enough time to enjoy a meal or snack without work interruptions if possible.

- When eating while socializing or conducting business, make it a point to alternately shift your focus from eating to the conversation.

- Be aware of the effects of alcohol on your ability to eat mindfully.

- Allowing the serving size or how much others are eating determine how much you'll eat can lead to overeating. Check in with your hunger and fullness levels to decide when to stop.

- Since meals tend to take longer at social events, you may need to have your plate removed or put your napkin on it when you're satisfied to avoid nibbling unconsciously.

If you're used to eating on autopilot, mindful eating may feel a little awkward at first. Like other strategies you've learned in this book, it becomes more natural with practice. By choosing to eat every bite with intention and attention, you'll find yourself eating less while experiencing more enjoyment. Look at what happened when Ted tried it:

I've been known to finish a bag of potato chips while watching football. Afterward I barely remember eating them, except that I feel stuffed and my blood sugar is sky high.

My wife and I went to an afternoon baseball game, and, while walking in, we smelled kettle corn. We both love that combination of sweet and salty popcorn, so I automatically got in line to buy a large bag. As I waited, I realized I wasn't even hungry yet, and, since the game would go on for hours, there was really no rush. So we went to our seats instead. By the fifth inning, we were both starting to get a little hungry. I reminded myself that when I'm only a little hungry, I only need a little food, so I bought the small bag of kettle corn to share with my wife. When I got back to my seat, I ate just one kernel at a time, savoring every bite. After a while, I noticed myself starting to get bored eating it that way and I wanted to shovel it by the handful like I used to. That made me laugh! What was the point of shoveling the popcorn just to get through it? I closed the bag, put it under my seat, and focused on the game instead. When I checked my blood sugar before dinner that evening, it was slightly above target but not sky high, like it would have been if I had eaten mindlessly.

Staying focused and fully present in the moment makes you aware of what you're thinking, feeling, and experiencing. This is what it means to truly love what you eat. Once you've experienced the pleasure of eating mindfully, become more mindful during other activities too. Use intention and attention in your conversations, work, walks—no matter what you're doing. Living fully in the moment allows you to listen and trust your innate wisdom, increasing your effectiveness and contentment in everything you do.

CHAPTER 14

Care:
Staying Healthy

This "Care" chapter explores ways to stay well by taking charge of your health beyond the day-to-day management of your blood glucose. As we look at the lab tests, consultations, and other preventive steps you can take to stay as healthy as possible, try not to get so focused on *what* to do that you lose sight of *why*. Ultimately, the reason for all of this is to seek optimal health.

Optimal health is the best health you can attain in the present, given your current level of understanding, effort, and circumstances, and it includes wellness of your body, mind, heart, and spirit. Optimal health is not perfect health; like it or not, you have prediabetes or diabetes, and perhaps you have other medical issues and life challenges to deal with. Optimal health cannot be defined by a lab result or achieved by checking a box, because it's a personal experience. It's not a destination but a dynamic, changing landscape. As you take charge of your diabetes and become more mindful, your personal definition of optimal health may evolve and expand.

Why Does Uncontrolled Diabetes Cause Problems?

Understanding the potential problems caused by uncontrolled diabetes and why they occur is essential for knowing the steps you can take now to prevent and screen for them so that you can stay as healthy as possible. Here's the simplest way to think about what causes these problems: when excess glucose travels through your body day after day, it begins to make tissues sticky; imagine a film of sugar coating your arteries, veins, and organs. In addition, high blood pressure and abnormal lipids can damage the tissues too. This causes problems (called *complications*) that can be placed in three groups.

Microvascular Disease

As you probably figured out, since *micro* means "small" and *vascular* refers to "blood vessels," *microvascular disease* affects the tiny blood vessels in your body. These tiny blood vessels are weakened by excess glucose floating in the bloodstream. Areas that are particularly prone to problems when these tiny vessels are damaged include the eyes, the kidneys, and the nerves in the feet and other parts of the body.

Retinopathy. When the blood vessels in the area called the *retina*, at the back of the eye, are damaged by diabetes, they can leak or rupture. This condition, called *retinopathy*, is the leading cause of vision loss in the United States (CDC 2011).

Nephropathy. Damage to the small vessels in the kidneys can cause them to leak protein into the urine, eventually causing scarring and other problems that prevent the kidneys from filtering the blood properly (called *nephropathy*). If this impaired kidney function (also called impaired renal function) worsens to the point where substances build up to dangerous levels in the blood, a machine will have to filter the blood, which is called *dialysis*. A kidney transplant may also be needed. Diabetes is the leading cause of kidney disease in the United States (ibid.).

Neuropathy. *Neuropathy* affects the ability of nerves to send and receive signals. Neuropathy in the feet can cause intense pain, burning, and sensitivity to touch. As the nerve function declines, the inability to sense pain, temperature, or even the feet touching the ground can develop. The loss of these protective sensations causes a series of problems that can result in injury, infections, and difficulty walking.

While neuropathy most commonly affects the feet, it can occur in other areas, like the stomach, where it slows down digestion (called *gastroparesis*), and the penis, where it can lead to sexual dysfunction and impotence.

Macrovascular Disease

Macrovascular disease affects the medium and large arteries in your body, including the coronary arteries, which are the vessels that take blood to the heart muscle; the cerebral arteries, which carry blood to the brain; and the peripheral (distant) arteries, which carry blood to the legs and feet. Uncontrolled diabetes accelerates the development of atherosclerosis in these blood vessels. Plaques, which are mounds of lipid material, cells, and calcium, build up in the inner wall of the blood vessel. These plaques get larger over time, gradually decreasing the flow of blood. The plaques can rupture, triggering the formation of a blood clot that completely blocks blood flow.

Coronary heart disease (CHD). When there's blockage in the coronary arteries, you may have symptoms like chest pain (called *angina*) or shortness of breath. A heart attack occurs when an area of heart muscle dies from lack of blood flow.

Cerebrovascular disease. A stroke is when an area of the brain doesn't get enough blood flow. The area of the brain affected will determine the symptoms, such as loss of speech or paralysis of one or more areas of the body.

Peripheral vascular disease (PVD). If the tissues in your leg don't get enough blood flow, you may have pain when you walk (called *claudication*). If the blood supply is completely blocked, the tissue can die, sometimes requiring amputation.

Impaired Immunity and Healing

Uncontrolled diabetes decreases the body's ability to fight off infection and impairs its ability to heal. As a result, people with diabetes may have a harder time recovering from viral illnesses, like colds and the flu, and infections, like pneumonia. They may also have delayed healing after both minor and serious injuries and surgeries. In addition, they may be more prone to *periodontal* (gum) disease in the mouth, which is now known to increase inflammation in the body and increase the risk of heart disease.

Strategies: What You Can Do to Stay Healthy

In addition to eating mindfully, being physically active, checking your blood glucose regularly, and taking medications as prescribed, there are a number of actions you can take to stay healthy and catch problems as early as possible.

Don't smoke. Smoking is known to increase microvascular and macrovascular disease. Ask for help quitting if needed; many programs and medications are available to help.

Have flu and pneumonia shots. Get a flu shot every year. You also need at least one pneumonia shot (also called a *pneumococcal vaccine*); some people also need a booster shot, so ask your primary care provider.

Check your feet. Check your feet thoroughly every day for problems like numbness, tingling, redness, swelling, tenderness, open sores, cracks, discolored skin, areas that feel hot to the touch, and sore toenails. They could be signs of infection, decreased circulation, or other complications, so call your health care professional that day and make sure you are seen within twenty-four hours.

Track your test results and visits. Download a diabetes care card from www.diabetesandmindfuleating.com. You may also find electronic programs online that will make it convenient for you to track and share information about your diabetes care.

Be prepared for your appointments. Take your medications, glucose meter, blood glucose log, and diabetes care card or program with you to all of your visits. Write down your questions and concerns ahead of time, and share them at the beginning of the visit so that your provider will be sure to leave enough time to address them.

Keep your weight stable. Changes in your weight can affect your blood glucose, medication dosage, and risk for complications. If your weight is rising, you'll need to make adjustments to your eating and physical activity. See your physician, dietitian, and exercise specialist for help.

Manage your cholesterol. High LDL cholesterol, low HDL cholesterol, and high triglycerides are also associated with macrovascular disease, so have your lipid panel checked annually (or according to your health care professional's recommendations) and treated as indicated. You may need to change your diet (see chapter 11), increase your exercise, see a specialist, start medications, or some combination.

Control your blood pressure. High blood pressure increases the risk of atherosclerosis, retinopathy, and nephropathy. The blood pressure goal for people with diabetes is 130/80 or less (or as advised by your health care professional) (AACE 2007a). If your blood pressure is elevated (*hypertension*), you may be advised to exercise, decrease the sodium in your diet, and lose weight. If it remains elevated, medications will be prescribed.

Limit your sodium intake. Most nutrition experts recommend a daily maximum of less than 2,300 mg of sodium. In 2010 the USDA recommended a reduction of sodium intake to 1,500 mg for African-Americans and people with hypertension or diabetes.

Follow sick-day guidelines. When you're ill, your blood glucose can become unstable. Infection, fever, loss of appetite, nausea, vomiting, and inactivity may cause it to be either too high or too low. Before you get sick, refer to the sick-day guidelines in chapter 18 and talk with your provider or diabetes educator to help you manage your diabetes during periods of illness.

Ask about preventive medications. Ask your primary care provider if you should be on preventive metformin, aspirin, medications for your kidneys, statins, or supplements.

Screen for eye disease. You need to see an ophthalmologist or qualified optometrist yearly for a thorough eye exam. During the exam, the doctor will dilate your pupils or take a photograph to view the retina at the back of the eye to see any sign of problems with the small blood vessels and other problems related to diabetes.

Take care of your teeth. Periodontal (gum) disease is an inflammatory process that is accelerated by and can cause elevated blood glucose. In addition, periodontal disease increases the risk of heart disease. Brush your teeth and floss regularly, and see your dentist or dental hygienist twice a year.

Talk to your health care team about your feelings. With any chronic illness, problems like depression and anxiety are relatively common. Share your feelings and concerns with your team and ask for help in coping with stress and other problems associated with having diabetes.

See your doctor before pregnancy. If you are a woman of childbearing age, see your health care provider to discuss preconception diabetes management.

Continue to learn. Take advantage of new learning opportunities available in your area, such as exercise groups, diabetes classes, support groups, or nonprofit and community events that support people with diabetes. Staying healthy requires an investment of time, money, and effort, but costs much less than coping with a complication.

How to Catch Problems Early

Many of the complications described previously do not cause noticeable symptoms until the problems are serious. Since an important goal of diabetes care is to prevent or lessen problems, a number of recommended evaluations, tests, and screenings are available to try to catch these problems as early as possible, and there are steps you can take to decrease your risks.

Diabetes Checkups

A diabetes checkup is recommended on initial diagnosis and every three to six months, depending on how stable your diabetes is. This visit is usually with your primary care provider unless you see an endocrinologist for your routine diabetes care. (Note: you should also schedule an annual complete physical to prevent, identify, and treat other conditions and to address other ways to achieve optimal health in addition to caring for your diabetes.)

During your diabetes checkup, you and your primary care provider will review your diet, physical activity, current medications, blood glucose log, and lab results. This is also a time to address any problems, concerns, or questions you have. Your provider will check your vital signs, order appropriate lab tests, and refer you to specialists as needed.

At your annual diabetes checkups, your provider will also conduct a focused examination to check for signs of problems, possibly looking at the backs of your eyes (called a funduscopic exam); feeling your thyroid gland; checking your skin, especially any insulin injection sites; checking your legs and feet; and checking your pulses and reflexes. The doctor may test your peripheral nerves by moving your toes while your eyes are closed to see if you can tell what position they are in, touching the side of your foot with a tuning fork to test your ability to detect vibration, and touching you lightly with a thin fiber called a *monofilament* to see if you can feel it.

Lab Work

Laboratory testing provides information about diabetes control, monitors other risk factors, and screens for early signs of complications.

A1C. A blood test called *hemoglobin A1c* (or HbA1c or A1C) is a way to examine your average blood glucose control over several months. This test will be done at diagnosis and two to four times a year, depending on how stable your blood glucose has been. The goal is usually an A1C of less than 7 percent because this has been shown to reduce microvascular complications (ADA 2011), but your care team may recommend a different goal for you. If your A1C is elevated, you and your team will review your current plan to see if medication changes or consultations with a diabetes educator, dietitian, or specialist are needed. You may also decide to renew your efforts to eat mindfully, be physically active, and test your blood glucose regularly.

Lipid panel. You will have your cholesterol panel checked once a year, more often if you have high cholesterol or cardiovascular disease (CVD). As a reminder, the goals for people with diabetes are:

- LDL: less than 100 mg/dL or less than 70 mg/dL if you have CVD.

- HDL: greater than 40 mg/dL in men and greater than 50 mg/dL in women

- Triglycerides: less than 150 mg/dL

If your tests are above these goals, you may need to change your diet (see chapter 11), increase your exercise, see a specialist, start medications, or try some combination of these tactics (AACE 2007b).

Screening for kidney disease. Your kidneys become less efficient as you get older; having diabetes, high blood pressure, or both speeds up the decline. In addition, some medications used to treat diabetes can affect the kidneys. When kidney function is declining, the kidneys leak small amounts of protein (*albumin*) into the urine; this is called *microalbuminuria*. You should have a yearly urine test for microalbumin to be sure that you are losing fewer than 30 milligrams of protein per gram of urine (ibid.). You will also have a yearly blood test for *creatinine* (Cr), which is a waste product; the results of this test are used to estimate the *glomerular filtration rate* (GFR) to tell how well your kidneys are removing wastes from the blood. If the microalbumin level, creatinine, or both are elevated, you may need adjustments to your diabetes care plan to be sure your diabetes and blood pressure are well controlled. You may also be placed on additional medications to protect your kidneys and referred to a diabetes educator to help you with your diabetes, a nephrologist for additional evaluation, or a dietitian for possible dietary changes for protection of your kidneys.

Your Health Care Team

You are the captain of your health care team. You'll want to carefully select the members of your team based on their skill, knowledge, and ability to communicate regularly and clearly with you.

Primary care provider. Your primary care provider is usually a family physician, internist, nurse practitioner, or physician's assistant who provides preventive care and regular diabetes checkups and helps coordinate your care with the rest of your team. You'll see your primary care provider annually for a complete physical, every three to six months for a diabetes checkup, and as needed for questions, concerns, new symptoms, and illnesses. Your provider will order the appropriate tests, write your prescriptions, and refer you to specialists when needed.

Diabetes educator. Your certified diabetes educator (CDE) helps you learn about and self-manage your diabetes. A CDE might be a registered nurse, registered dietitian, pharmacist, physical therapist, exercise physiologist, social worker, psychologist, or any other qualified health professional who has completed advanced training in caring for diabetes. Ideally, you'll meet with a CDE when you are initially diagnosed with diabetes and yearly thereafter. At these appointments you'll learn about diabetes, including how to test your blood glucose and analyze patterns, how to recognize symptoms of high and low blood glucose, what to do when you are sick, how to take your diabetes medications, and what your lab tests mean. You'll also download the results from your glucose meter and verify its accuracy. You'll discuss how you are coping with having diabetes and any other questions, problems, or concerns you have.

Registered dietitian or nutritionist. A registered dietitian (RD) or a nutritionist will help you learn about food, nutrition, and lifestyle changes. You will typically see this professional when you are initially diagnosed with either prediabetes or diabetes and two or more times each year thereafter as needed for medical nutrition therapy. This person will help you learn more about your diet and how to eat healthier, learn about carbohydrate counting and meal planning, and understand your blood glucose and how the foods you eat affect it. This clinician will recommend changes in your diet to minimize your risk from other conditions, such as managing high cholesterol or lowering the sodium in your diet for hypertension. This person can also help you learn how to balance food with medications and activity, make a sick-day meal plan, and plan for eating out and handling special events.

Ophthalmologist. An ophthalmologist is a physician who specializes in eye health. You will see this doctor within a year of diagnosis and annually after that. At these appointments, you will have a detailed eye exam, including an examination of the retina to detect eye diseases associated with diabetes.

Endocrinologist. An endocrinologist is a physician who specializes in diabetes. You may be referred to an endocrinologist if you have unexplained hyperglycemia or hypoglycemia; poorly controlled diabetes, as indicated by an A1C higher than 8 for six to twelve months; or other chronic medical conditions, such as heart disease or kidney disease; or if you need information on how to use an insulin pump or other special diabetes-related technology.

Podiatrist. A podiatrist specializes in foot health, so you may be referred for new or ongoing problems with your feet. Examples include a history of foot problems, such as injury, peripheral vascular disease, amputation, or deformities; new sores, cuts, wounds, ingrown toenails, or calluses; or symptoms like pain, burning, or problems with your shoes; as well as for routine foot care if you have difficulty safely cutting your own toenails due to hand strength, vision, mobility, or other problems.

Pharmacist. Your pharmacist will explain how to take your medications correctly and safely and how to look for drug interactions with your other medications, and will answer any questions you may have. This person may suggest lower-cost substitutions when appropriate. Additionally, your pharmacist can advise you about over-the-counter medications. Many are also knowledgeable about supplements and complementary medicine, so be sure to tell the pharmacist all of the vitamins, minerals, supplements, and anything else you are taking.

Dentist. See your dentist and dental hygienist every six to twelve months to examine your teeth and gums for dental and periodontal disease and to have your teeth cleaned.

Exercise specialist. A personal trainer or exercise physiologist is a great addition to your team for setting up an individualized exercise program, learning how to use the gym or a specific piece of equipment, and providing motivation and accountability. Some exercise specialists are also CDEs or may have additional training in diabetes or cardiac disease.

Other specialists. Your other team players may also include a cardiologist to screen for and treat heart disease; a nephrologist for kidney problems; a smoking cessation counselor; a mental health counselor, social worker, psychologist, or therapist to help with the emotional challenges of having a chronic disease; and other specialists as determined by your team members.

CHAPTER 15

Nourish:
Fat Facts

This chapter explores the role of fat in your diet. Before we begin, pause to consider what you know, believe, and feel about consuming fat.

You're probably already aware that fat is important because of its link to cholesterol and heart disease. You may also know that a diet high in solid fat raises your cholesterol and risk of heart disease. But have you noticed that fat also affects your blood glucose management? Are you interested in learning more, or do you feel dread or boredom? Admittedly, fat can be a confusing topic because our understanding of the role of fat in the diet has changed radically over the last few decades. With all of this new information, it can be challenging to remember which types are beneficial and which types contribute to heart disease.

Fat-containing foods are still high on some people's "forbidden food" lists—a leftover from the low-fat diet craze. The thought of learning about fat can trigger the restrictive eating cycle and feelings of deprivation, shame, and guilt. Some people might notice that they would prefer to ignore or avoid this topic altogether.

The Big Picture

The intent of learning about nutrition isn't to restrict or perfect your diet. It's simply to provide information in a way that's easy to understand and remember so that you can mindfully choose what to eat. With fat, you might like Jenny's approach:

During my years of dieting, I felt guilty whenever I ate anything that wasn't low fat. I knew times had changed, but at first, the more I learned, the more confused and conflicted I felt. I decided to think of fat like money: I need it to survive and enjoy my life! To be healthy with diabetes, I also need to stay within my budget. Since I'm kind of a "numbers person," I thought, if grams of fat are dollars, I get to decide where I spend my money each day. To me, choosing unsaturated fats is an investment in my health, and saturated and trans fats are an expense. I find that I feel healthiest and happiest when I include both in my budget. I noticed that including a little fat in my meals and snacks leaves me feeling more satisfied, and my blood sugar is better.

Jenny's budget analogy might be helpful for you too because it provides flexibility, perspective, and wisdom for making decisions. Ideally, you'd set your budget based on the latest research and then decide how you prefer to spend your money. As with money, everyone chooses to spend it a little differently. Even if you aren't a "numbers person," you may want to track your "spending" for a couple of weeks to increase your awareness about the amount and types of fats you eat.

Let's begin by describing how fat affects your body, the risk of heart disease, cholesterol levels, and diabetes management. We'll then explain what you need to know about the different types of fat and provide some tips to help you make decisions for yourself.

Fat and Your Health

Fats are important to your health for many reasons:

- One gram of dietary fat provides your body with nine calories to use or store as energy. For comparison, carbohydrates and protein each have four calories per gram, so fat is considered "calorie dense."

- Fat is essential for growth and development (especially brain development during childhood).

- Fat is necessary for the absorption and transportation of vitamins A, D, E, and K.

- Fat helps maintain healthy skin and hair.

- Fat increases satiety (satisfaction and fullness).

- Fat gives food flavor and texture.

- Polyunsaturated fat improves cholesterol levels and reduces cardiovascular risk.

- Omega-3 fatty acids in fish oil decrease the risk of heart disease, stroke, and overall mortality.

- Excessive intake of saturated fat, trans fat, and cholesterol is associated with heart disease and stroke.

Fat and Heart Disease

The relationship between fat intake and cardiovascular disease is important because, when you have diabetes, you are two to four times more likely to suffer from heart disease and stroke than someone without diabetes. In fact, two out of three people with type 1 or type 2 diabetes will die from these causes (CDC 2011). While these are frightening statistics, awareness and knowledge empower you to minimize your personal risk.

There are many known risk factors for heart disease and stroke. While some of them are beyond your control—family history, age, and gender—other risk factors, including smoking, high blood pressure, diabetes, obesity, physical inactivity, and high cholesterol, are under your influence. Therefore, quitting smoking; exercising regularly; and managing your blood pressure, diabetes, weight, and cholesterol are all meaningful steps that you can take to live a longer, healthier life. Be sure to speak with your health care professional about your personal risk factors and the specific steps you should consider. This chapter focuses on the changes you can make in your diet that lower your risk.

Fat and Diabetes

Knowledge about fat is also important when you have diabetes because including a moderate amount of healthy fats in your diet can help stabilize your blood glucose (Gannon and Nuttall 2006). How? Eating fat with meals and snacks is a flavorful, low-carbohydrate way to satisfy hunger. Fat is satiating; in other words, it fills you up and keeps you full so that you may eat fewer carbohydrates overall. In addition, eating carbohydrates along with 5 or 10 grams of fat slows down absorption of glucose (Harding et al. 2001). Examples of foods with 5 grams of healthy fat include one tablespoon of peanut butter, two to three thin slices of avocado, or eight large olives. Other studies have shown that when people eat one ounce of nuts a day, they have improved blood glucose control (Wien et al. 2010; Jenkins et al. 2006). Eating nuts also decreases the risk of developing diabetes in the first place (Jiang et al. 2002).

What Are Fats Anyway?

What we commonly call "fats" are actually lipids, which include fats, oils, cholesterol, and triglycerides. Numerous health authorities recommend that your total fat intake be in the range of 20 to 35 percent of your total calories. (See typical serving sizes in the following table.) However, research has shown that the total amount of fat in the diet isn't really linked with disease; what really matters are the *types* of fat you eat. That's why Jenny thinks about her budget in terms of investments and expenses. Let's take a closer look at each type.

Fat

Typical Serving Sizes	
Margarine, butter	1 teaspoon
Mayonnaise	1 teaspoon
Nuts (almonds, peanuts, walnuts, etc.)	6–10
Reduced fat mayonnaise or margarine	1 tablespoon
Reduced fat salad dressing	2 tablespoon
Salad dressing	1 tablespoon
Sour cream	2 tablespoon

Figure 15.1

Cholesterol

Cholesterol plays an important functional role in your body, but too much can contribute to your risk of heart disease. Cholesterol comes from two sources: it's made in your liver and consumed in your diet. Your cholesterol levels are primarily hereditary and partly dietary. Your liver manufactures cholesterol, which is necessary for building cell membranes and nerve tissue, helping produce necessary hormones for body regulation, and producing bile acids for digestion. Other animals manufacture cholesterol for these same reasons; therefore dietary cholesterol is found in the animal products you may eat, such as meat, poultry, egg yolks, cheese, whole milk, and other whole-milk dairy products. (These animal products also contain saturated fat, which, as you'll see next, also increases cholesterol levels.)

For some people, high cholesterol levels and heart disease run in the family; their bodies may be genetically programmed to manufacture too much cholesterol. Others manufacture the right amount of cholesterol but eat too much cholesterol, saturated fat, and trans fat in their diets, raising their blood cholesterol levels and putting themselves at increased risk of heart disease.

Knowing your cholesterol level is necessary for evaluating whether you are at increased risk of heart disease, but the total cholesterol doesn't tell the whole story. Cholesterol is transported in different forms, which have different effects.

LDL. *Low-density lipoproteins* (LDL) are considered "bad" because they are sticky and likely to form fatty deposits and plaque on the walls of your arteries, which leads to blockage. Eating polyunsaturated and monounsaturated fats (olive, peanut, and canola oils) may help lower your LDL levels. Here's a way to remember this: *LDL* means *lousy* cholesterol, so the *lower*, the better. A healthy person's LDL level should be less than 130 mg/dL. A person with diabetes should maintain an LDL level of less than 100 mg/dL. Anyone with cardiovascular disease should aim for less than 70 mg/dL (AACE 2007b).

HDL. *High-density lipoproteins* (HDL) are considered "good" because they help carry away cholesterol that is stuck to the walls of the arteries. Regular physical activity and exercise can raise your levels of this "good" cholesterol. Here's a way to remember this: *HDL* means *healthy* cholesterol, so the *higher*, the better. A high level of HDL is associated with a lower incidence of heart disease. An HDL level of more than 40 mg/dL in men and 50 mg/dL in women is optimal.

Authorities recommend a cholesterol intake of fewer than 300 milligrams daily. People with diabetes or a personal or family history of elevated cholesterol levels or heart disease need to be even more cautious about eating high-cholesterol foods and saturated fats. Take a look at the suggestions at the end of this chapter or consult a dietitian to help you determine how to change your diet. If your total and LDL cholesterol levels remain high despite following a diet low in cholesterol and saturated fat and exercising regularly, medications may be necessary to lower your cholesterol to safe levels. Discuss this with your health care professional.

Triglycerides

Triglycerides are another form in which fat is transported through the blood. Triglyceride levels above 150 mg/dL are considered a risk factor for heart disease. Elevated triglyceride levels can be the result of eating meals high in carbohydrates, calories, or fat; having diabetes; being overweight; drinking excess alcohol; or having an inherited lipid or pancreatic disorder. Very high levels can have other serious medical complications, so treatment with diet (including omega-3 fatty acids) and medication (if needed) is warranted.

Saturated and Unsaturated Fats

Fats (also called "fatty acids") are made of long chains of carbon atoms that like to bond with hydrogen atoms.

Saturated Fat

Saturated fat is typically solid at room temperature. This solid fat is found in animal products, including meat and meat products, dairy products, egg yolks, and butter. Tropical oils, like palm, palm kernel, and coconut oils, are also saturated; they may be found in candy, snack products, and movie popcorn.

Saturated fats raise blood cholesterol, which increases the risk of heart disease. Here's an easy way to remember this: *saturated* fat is *solid* at room temperature and *sits* in your arteries.

The American Heart Association recommends limiting your intake of saturated fat to less than 7 percent of your total daily calories (Lichtenstein et al. 2006).

Unsaturated Fat

Unsaturated fats are oils because they are liquid at room temperature. These "healthy fats" are typically found in plant products and fish.

- Polyunsaturated fat is primarily found in oils: safflower, sunflower, corn, sesame seed, flaxseed, soybean, and cottonseed. Fish is also an excellent source.

- Monounsaturated fat sources include canola oil, olive oil, and peanut oil. Here's a helpful way to remember them: good COP (*canola, olive, peanut*). Avocados, nuts, olives, and peanut butter are also good sources of monounsaturated fats.

Replacing unhealthy saturated fats in your diet with healthy unsaturated fats can help reduce total cholesterol and prevent heart disease.

Omega-3 Fatty Acids

Omega-3 fatty acids are a type of polyunsaturated fats. Health benefits from omega-3s include decreased risk of arrhythmias (abnormal heartbeats) and decreased triglyceride levels. Omega-3s also slow the buildup of plaque in the arteries and lower blood pressure slightly.

Good sources of omega-3 fatty acids include cold-water fish (mackerel, salmon, tuna), flaxseed and its oil, canola oil, walnuts and their oil, and soybeans and their oil. The American Heart Association recommends that most adults eat two 4-ounce servings of fatty fish each week to consume an adequate amount of omega-3s (Lichtenstein et al. 2006). If you have a history of heart disease, the American Heart Association recommends one serving of fish daily (Kris-Etherton et al. 2002).

Trans Fat

Another type of fat, trans fat, primarily results from man-made processes that alter unsaturated fats. Food manufacturers make trans fat by bubbling hydrogen gas into liquid vegetable oils, which causes hydrogen bonds to form to make the liquid solid or semisolid. Eating trans fat increases your LDL levels, decreases your HDL levels, and raises your risk of heart disease and stroke.

- Trans fats are found in many foods, especially fried foods; baked goods, including pastries, pie crusts, biscuits, pizza dough, cookies, and crackers; and stick margarines.

- Trans fats are listed on the nutrition label when there is half a gram or more per serving. They will also be found in the ingredient list as hydrogenated or partially hydrogenated oils, even when there is less than half a gram in each serving. The closer to the beginning of the list an ingredient appears, the more of it the product contains.

The American Heart Association recommends limiting the amount of trans fats you eat to less than 1 percent of your total daily calories (Lichtenstein et al. 2006).

How to Wisely Invest Your Fat Intake

The following tips will help you get the most value from your fat.

Decrease Your Intake of Saturated Fat

- Use liquid oils instead of solid fat whenever possible.

- Select leaner cuts of beef and pork (they often have the words "round" or "loin" in the name), trim visible fat, and remove the skin from chicken before cooking. Choose ground beef labeled "lean" (ideally less than 10 percent fat). Drain excess fat (or rinse with hot water in a colander) before adding additional ingredients.

- Try meatless meals using vegetable sources of protein, like beans and soy.

- Use low-fat or nonfat (skim) versions of your favorite dairy products. Use small amounts of cheese; grate and sprinkle it for flavor rather than using large chunks or sauces.

Choose Unsaturated Fats

- Buy or make salad dressings with vegetable, olive, or canola oil. Also, use these oils in place of butter or lard when cooking.

- Use a thin spread of avocado or guacamole in place of mayonnaise or butter on a sandwich.

- Olives add a flavorful and beneficial dose of fat to pastas, salads, and other dishes.

- Peanut butter is an old standby: high in fat but satisfying in small amounts. Read the label to check for added sugars.

- Tree nuts, like almonds and walnuts, have additional health benefits. They can make a great snack and add nice flavor to pasta dishes and salads.

Eat More Omega-3 Fatty Acids

- The omega-3 fatty acids in fish oil decrease the risk of heart disease, stroke, and overall mortality. Try to eat at least two 4-ounce servings of fish each week.

- Fatty fish, such as salmon, tuna, rainbow trout, herring, mackerel, and wild oysters have the highest levels of omega-3s.

- If you don't like fish, consider taking fish oil capsules (one gram daily) and increasing your intake of flaxseed, canola oil, and walnuts.

Watch Trans Fats

- Look for trans fat on the "Nutrition Facts" label and check the ingredient list for hydrogenated or partially hydrogenated oil.

- Ask whether your favorite restaurants use trans fat for frying, cooking, or baking.

Reduce Your Total Fat Intake

- Prepare or order foods that are grilled, roasted, baked, boiled, or braised instead of fried or sautéed.

- Use less butter, oil, mayonnaise, cream cheese, salad dressing, sauces, and toppings.

- Ask for your salad dressing and sauces on the side. Dip the tip of the tines of your fork in the dressing before you spear your salad; you'll get a little flavor with every bite but a lot less fat than you would if it were poured on.

- Spray your pans with cooking spray instead of coating them with fats and oils.

- Try baked tortilla chips, whole-wheat pita bread, and whole-grain crackers with healthy dips and toppings, like hummus, in place of higher-fat chips and crackers.

- Use moderation for the higher-fat foods you really love.

Whew! That was a lot of information. To put this into perspective, let's take a look at how Jenny uses her budget:

I invest most of my fat budget in healthy polyunsaturated and monoun- saturated fats. Now, when I read a nutrition label, I look for the grams of fat and saturated fat per serving to see how much it will cost. The "four really" test—Do I really, really, really, really want it?— helps me decide whether it's worth it.

CHAPTER 16

Live:
Increase Your Strength

This chapter's title may conjure up images of body building, but the real purpose of strength training is to lower your blood glucose, decrease insulin resistance, increase your metabolism, and help you become stronger and healthier day by day.

Why Bother?

Building muscle tissue and increasing your strength has many benefits, including:

- Improving your glucose metabolism (Sigal et al. 2004)

- Lowering your A1C (Sigal et al. 2006)

- Increasing your ability to function in your daily life

- Enabling you to lift a heavy object and repeatedly lift a lighter object

- Maintaining or boosting your metabolism by increasing your muscle mass

- Minimizing the loss of your lean body mass while you are losing weight

- Contributing to a leaner, more-toned appearance

- Helping prevent age-related decreases in your muscle mass (Lemmer et al. 2000)

- Reducing the risk of overuse injuries by balancing the strength of opposing muscle groups

- Decreasing lower-back pain by strengthening the core of your body

- Increasing your bone mineral density to prevent or treat osteoporosis (Maddalozzo et al. 2007)

- Lowering your blood pressure and cholesterol levels

- Helping you appreciate the capacity of your body to meet the demands you place on it

What You Need to Know

Strength training, also called *resistance training*, is exercise that makes your muscles work harder than they're accustomed to. As a result, the muscle fibers become larger and stronger. To build your muscles, you can lift your own body weight against gravity (like doing sit-ups or push-ups), work against resistance (like pushing an immobile object or pushing and pulling rubber tubing), or lift weights (like using free weights or exercise equipment designed for that purpose). Michelle shares her story about introducing strength training to her exercise routine:

> *For several years, I enjoyed walking for exercise. When I learned about the benefits of strength training, I decided to add some floor exercises to my routine. The first time I tried to do a push-up, I couldn't even do one. I felt discouraged and gave up. Later, it dawned on me that the fact that I couldn't do a single push-up was exactly why I needed to try!*
>
> *Every other day I tried to do push-ups again. I imagined my muscles saying, "For some reason, she wants us to lift her off the floor instead of just let her lie here. We'd better get to work." On the opposite days, I could imagine my muscle fibers getting stronger. If I gave up, said, "I can't do push-ups," and never tried again, my muscles would go back to the way they were. Eventually I was able to do push-ups—but I was even happier when I realized that I could easily lift my own luggage in and out of the*

overhead bin. Now I often share my "one push-up principle" to help moti-vate people to get started. Strength training isn't a matter of can and can't. It's a matter of if and when.

About 25 percent of your metabolism (your daily caloric need) is driven by the amount of muscle tissue you have (ACSM 2006). Muscle is more meta-bolically active than fat; the more muscle you have, the more fuel you burn, even when you are at rest.

In fact, most of the age-related slowing of metabolism is due to lack of physical activity and loss of muscle tissue. Studies have shown a 5 percent decline in metabolism each decade throughout adulthood and a 25 percent decline in muscle function by age sixty-five (ibid.). This is why you may feel as if you eat the way you did when you were younger but gain weight more easily.

The effects of yo-yo dieting compound this problem. Every time you dras-tically decrease your calorie intake, you lose muscle, not just fat, if you aren't exercising regularly. Once you abandon the diet and resume eating the way you previously did, you'll quickly regain fat but not the muscle you lost. As a result, your metabolism will be even slower, often leading to even more weight gain and a higher body fat percentage, which makes you more prone to diabe-tes, atherosclerosis, and other chronic diseases.

Be Strong, Be Healthy

There are two ways to look at muscle fitness. *Muscular strength* is the ability of a muscle to exert maximal force for a brief period. This is how much weight a person can lift once (for example, lifting a bag of dog food out of the trunk). *Muscular endurance* is the ability of a muscle or group of muscles to perform many repetitions against resistance (for example, lifting a small child into the air repeatedly while playing). Resistance training will help you build both muscular strength and muscular endurance. Fortunately, you can maintain and even gain muscle at any age.

If you are trying to manage your weight, strength training will help pre-vent muscle loss that would otherwise occur as your body weight decreases. This is important because maintaining your muscle mass is crucial for regu-lating glucose levels and maintaining an active metabolism. In addition, resis-tance exercise, such as weight training, burns calories and lowers your blood glucose *during* exercise. Resistance exercise also improves glucose absorption by the muscle cells, therefore lowering your blood glucose level *after* your strength-training session is over.

Since there are remarkable changes happening in your muscles, you'll notice your strength improve fairly quickly. Don't concern yourself about getting too bulky or muscle bound from strength training. Most people don't have the genetic capability or the time to gain that much muscle. Women, with their relative lack of the male hormone testosterone, are very unlikely to bulk up. In fact, as muscle mass increases and body fat decreases, you'll look leaner and lose girth, even if your weight doesn't change.

Most important, keep in mind that while the changes may or may not be evident on the scale, as your ratio of muscle to fat increases, you're becoming stronger and healthier, lowering your blood glucose and decreasing insulin resistance.

Getting Started

Consult your physician before starting an exercise program. Consider seeking the advice of an exercise professional for a specific fitness prescription and instruction. Follow proper technique and form to decrease the chance of injury and optimize your results. This really helped Marcus and his wife, Gina:

> We joined our local YMCA, but I just used the treadmill and Gina only took group classes at first. We finally arranged a session with a personal trainer, who showed us how to use all of the equipment and designed strength-training programs for each of us. I feel we're really getting our money's worth at the gym now.

It's important to prepare your muscles for strength training by doing a brief warm-up first. It's better to warm up the muscle groups you'll be working than to do a generalized cardiorespiratory warm-up, such as walking. For example, if you plan to do an upper-body strength-training workout, warm up the chest, back, shoulder, arm, and core muscles; if you're doing a lower-body workout, warm up the lower back, buttocks, hips, and legs. The simplest way to do this is to simulate the exercises you plan to do, without using any weights.

You can vary strength-training exercises by how much weight you lift or move, how much resistance you push or pull against, how long you hold a weight up against gravity, and how many times you repeat the exercise during a session. This last variable is usually measured in reps and sets. *Rep* stands for "repetition": lifting a weight or doing an exercise once. A *set* is a certain number of repetitions. For example, if you lifted a hand weight ten times and then rested and repeated, you did two sets of ten reps.

During your strength-training session, start off doing only as many reps of the exercise as you can do comfortably, eventually working yourself up to a set of eight to fifteen reps (or hold for ten to thirty seconds, depending on the exercise). If you can't do at least eight reps, reduce the weight or resistance. If you can do more than fifteen reps, increase the weight or the resistance. As you practice, your body will get stronger to meet the demands you're placing on it. Gradually increase the number of reps, the amount of weight, or the number of sets, aiming for two to three sets for each exercise.

Do each exercise as slowly as possible, focusing your attention on the muscles you're using. Exhale slowly during the part of the exercise that requires the most effort. For example, during leg lifts, exhale while raising your leg and inhale while lowering it.

It takes just two sessions a week to begin to see results. It's important that you rest a muscle group for a minimum of forty-eight hours between weight-training sessions to allow the muscles to repair and become stronger. People who want to do strength training every day usually alternate between lower- and upper-body exercises, or work on even smaller groups of muscles. For general health and to increase muscular strength and endurance, training each muscle group properly even once a week is sufficient.

Simple Strength Training

There are many ways to build your strength. You can do this simple routine at home, in a hotel room, or even in your office without any equipment. It uses your body weight against the resistance of gravity to help you build muscle. You'll focus on your large muscles to get a great return on your investment.

Wall Squats

Muscles: Buttocks and legs

1. Stand with your back against a wall and your feet one thigh's length away from the wall.

2. Bend your knees and lower yourself as if you were going to sit down.

3. Press into the wall with your entire back while squeezing your buttocks and leg muscles. Eventually you'll be able to get your thighs parallel to the ground. Hold for as long as possible, aiming for ten to thirty seconds.

4. Repeat.

Modification: Use an exercise ball between your back and the wall for additional support. It's easiest to roll the ball down the wall to get into a sitting position.

Push-ups

Muscles: Chest, shoulders, arms, and upper back

At the Wall

1. Place your hands flat on a wall at shoulder height, ensuring that they are wider than shoulder width.

2. Place your feet far enough away from the wall that you can push yourself off the wall.

3. Bend your elbows and slowly bring your body closer to the wall again, keeping your chin lifted off your chest.

4. Repeat eight to fifteen times per set.

On Your Knees

1. While on all fours, with your knees directly under your hips and your hands slightly wider than shoulder width, bend your elbows, lowering your upper body toward the floor, and then press yourself back up. As you become stronger, move your knees farther behind your hips.

2. Repeat eight to fifteen times per set.

On Your Toes

1. Lie down on your stomach, positioning your hands under your shoulders, slightly wider than shoulder width.

2. Push your entire body off the ground while on your toes. Try to maintain a plank position by not allowing your hips to sag down or lift toward the ceiling.

3. Slowly raise and lower your entire body toward the ground.

4. Repeat eight to fifteen times per set. Alternatively, hold the plank position for ten to thirty seconds.

Superman

Muscles: Lower back

1. Lie face down on the floor with your arms straight out in front of you. Keep your neck in a neutral position by looking down at the floor a few inches ahead of you.

2. Lift your right arm and, if possible, left leg and hold for ten to thirty seconds per set.

3. Switch sides. As you get stronger, lift both legs and arms at the same time.

Modification: Position yourself comfortably on your hands and knees, with your back level and your neck in neutral position. Start by stretching your right arm out in front of you next to your right ear. If possible, straighten your left leg out behind you at the same time. Hold for ten to thirty seconds per set. Switch sides.

Leg Lifts

Muscles: Outer and inner thighs and buttocks

1. Lie on one side on the floor. Bend both legs 45 degrees. Place the arm that's on the floor under your head.

2. Lift your top leg about halfway as you tighten your muscles in your buttocks and leg.

3. Lift and lower your leg slowly eight to fifteen times per set. For added intensity, do not touch your top leg to your bottom leg.

4. Roll to the other side and repeat.

Bridge

Muscles: Buttocks, thighs, lower back, and abdominals

1. Lie on your back on the floor.

2. Bend your knees and place your feet hip-distance apart.

3. Tighten your buttocks and raise your hips off the floor, and then slowly lower them to the floor. To increase the intensity, do not lower your hips all the way down to the floor.

4. Repeat eight to fifteen times per set. Alternatively, hold for ten to thirty seconds per set.

Sit-ups

Muscles: Abdominals

1. Lie on your back on the floor.

2. Bend your knees and place your feet hip-distance apart.

3. Place your hands behind your head or cross your arms across your chest.

4. Keep your neck in neutral position (don't bring your chin toward your chest), and relax your arms and legs.

5. Tighten your abdominal muscles to lift your shoulder blades just off the floor, and then slowly lower down.

6. Repeat eight to fifteen times per set.

If doing repetitions with your hands across your chest or behind your head is too challenging, bring your hands to the backs of your thighs and gently pull your shoulders off the floor, keeping your chin neutral. Hold for eight to fifteen seconds, breathing normally (don't hold your breath!). Rest and repeat.

Fitness Rx: FITT Formula for More Strength

You can also build your strength by applying the FITT Formula to the exercises you do.

- *Frequency:* Two or more sessions per week

- *Intensity:* Two to three sets of eight to fifteen repetitions, or fifteen-to-thirty-second holds per exercise

- *Duration:* Typically about twenty to thirty minutes per session

- *Type:* Any activity that works against resistance, such as your body weight, rubber tubing, free weights, or exercise equipment

Keep It Interesting

- Consider purchasing other home exercise equipment, such as a weight bench or a home gym, or use cans of food, or milk jugs partially filled with sand or water if you enjoy the convenience and privacy of working out at home.

- A stability ball—a large, rubber exercise ball—is one of the most versatile and affordable pieces of exercise equipment. It's excellent for strength training (especially core strength), flexibility, balance, and coordination. You can do squats, sit-ups, push-ups, and numerous other exercises with the support of the ball.

- If the ball is the most versatile, a rubber exercise band or tubing is the most portable piece of resistance equipment. You can hook these long, wide rubber bands around your feet or wrists to provide resistance while doing various exercises. Tighten the band to increase the resistance as needed.

- Exercise in the water. Aquatic exercise enhances your cardiorespiratory fitness, while the resistance of the water increases your muscular strength and endurance. Water also provides buoyancy and support for your body, reducing stress and strain on your joints and muscles.

- Check your local community center or parks and recreation department for classes, or join a fitness center. Choose a convenient and comfortable place.

- Hire a qualified and experienced personal trainer. This person's expertise can help you develop a safe, efficient exercise program and keep you motivated to reach your fitness goals.

As you build new muscle, you'll find it easier to stabilize your blood glucose and maintain a healthier weight. Improving your muscular strength and endurance will increase your metabolism and help you function more fully in your life. For a limited investment in time, strength training pays big rewards.

PART 5

Letting Go

Some of us think holding on makes us strong, but sometimes it is letting go.

—Hermann Hesse

CHAPTER 17

Think:
How Much Do I Eat?

When you live in a land of abundance, deciding how much food you *need* to eat is critical for diabetes management and health. Just as important, when you eat the perfect amount of food, you'll feel satisfied—just right.

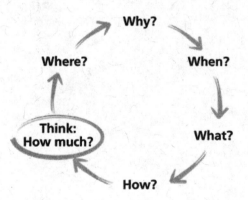

Figure 17.1

Just Right

Consider for a moment how you feel right after eating. When you're satisfied, you simply don't need anything else. You feel content, fulfilled, pleased, and even happy. How wonderful it is to feel good when you're finished eating.

It can be challenging too. You may eat past the point of satisfaction for many reasons: habits and learned behaviors, past dieting, and, often, not paying attention while you're eating. When you eat more than you need, you'll feel unnecessarily uncomfortable, your blood glucose may rise, and your body will have no choice but to store the excess as fat. Eating too much may cause you to have less energy and be less active. In the past, it may have also led to feelings of guilt, which usually led to even more overeating.

As you practice eating mindfully, with intention and attention, your awareness will change your perception of overeating. For example, when you're disconnected from hunger and fullness and you overeat for emotional reasons, it may actually feel good, at least temporarily. When you're aware and more connected, you'll feel physically uncomfortable and recognize that eating didn't meet your emotional needs very well.

To change those old patterns, you'll need to rediscover how great it feels when you don't overeat—and learn what to do on those occasions when you do. It's critical for you to tune in to your thoughts, feelings, and behaviors *without* judgment. You don't go through this process to punish yourself but to see what you can learn from the experience.

Compare teaching yourself to eat just the right amount of food to teaching a child to ride a bike. Do children learn easily when you get angry or criticize them for making mistakes? Will they feel like giving up if they're expected to ride perfectly right away? Will they want to try again if they're ashamed about falling off? Or do they learn best when you observe their actions, encourage each positive step they take, and offer gentle suggestions on ways to improve? Do they want to keep trying because you focus on how much they are progressing, not on what they do wrong? Will they feel encouraged when they notice it gets a little easier each time? Learning to stop eating when you're satisfied is exactly the same. You're most likely to learn when you're gentle, patient, encouraging, and optimistic with yourself throughout the process.

And, as with riding a bike, this process eventually becomes natural. Occasionally, something will throw you off balance, but because you've practiced and learned to make necessary adjustments and corrections, you'll keep cruising right along.

Enough Is Enough

As we've worked our way around the mindful eating cycle, you've learned numerous strategies to help you eat the amount of food your body needs. You learned that mindful eating requires intention and attention. Your intention is to meet your body's needs and to feel better when you're finished than you did when you started, in other words, satisfied. You pay attention to make it possible to eat less while enjoying your food more. Let's pick up where we left off and build on those strategies. We'll also use the mindful eating cycle to figure out why you overeat sometimes and how to quickly move back into instinctive eating. Please review figure 1.1.

How Full Am I?

Your awareness and the Hunger and Fullness Scale are your most useful tools for helping you determine when enough is enough. Just as you use your hunger level to let you know when to eat, you'll use your fullness level to let you know when you've had enough. Review figure 5.1.

Before you start eating, give yourself a hunger and fullness number, and decide what you want that number to be when you're finished. Estimate how much food you'll need to eat to reach that level of fullness. Prepare, serve, or order only as much as you think you'll need; if you were served too much, move the extra food aside. Before you start eating, visually or physically divide the food in half to create a "speed bump." Eat mindfully and check your fullness level when you hit that speed bump in the middle of eating, at the end of your meal, and again twenty to thirty minutes later.

Here are some questions you might ask yourself to help determine your level of fullness:

- *How does my stomach feel? Can I feel the food? Is there any discomfort or pain? Does my stomach feel stretched, full, or bloated?*

- *How does my body feel? Do I feel comfortable and content? Do my clothes feel tight? Is there any nausea or heartburn? Do I feel short of breath?*

- *How is my energy level? Do I feel energetic and ready for the next activity? Or am I sleepy, sluggish, tired, or lethargic?*

- *What do I feel like doing now?*

- *What's my blood glucose level?*

Based on your answers, determine your number on the Hunger and Fullness Scale.

Level 4 or lower. You're still a little hungry. You have several options:

- You could eat a little more; just a few bites may be all you need.

- You could wait a while to see whether you feel fuller; if not, you could eat a little more.

- You could stop eating for now. This is a great strategy if you plan to have dessert, if you'll eat again soon, or if you don't want to feel the food in your stomach, for example, before you exercise.

Level 5. You're satisfied and comfortable. You aren't hungry anymore yet don't feel the food in your body. You could eat more but don't need (or want) to. You may also notice that while you were eating, the flavor of the food went from fabulous to just okay as you became less hungry. It may have been harder to give food and eating your full attention. You feel light, energetic, and ready for your next activity. Where will you invest that energy? A lot more on this is coming up in chapter 21; in the meantime, just remember that the real purpose of eating is to fuel living.

Level 6. You're slightly full. You can feel the food in your stomach, but it's not unpleasant. When you're at level 5 or 6, you may want to move away from the table or move the food away from you to signal that you're finished. Pay close attention to this comfortable, contented feeling and try to remember it for next time.

Level 7 or higher. You feel somewhere between very full to sick. Picture your stomach as a balloon, as discussed in chapter 5. It can stretch far beyond its ideal capacity, but when it does, what is it pressing on or pushing out of the way? At level 7 or above, you think, *I ate too much! I bet my blood glucose will be above target.* You feel uncomfortable, regretful, and possibly sleepy and sluggish.

Notice that we intentionally used the word "regretful" instead of "guilty." What happens when you feel guilty about eating? Guilt is a powerful driver of the overeating cycle. Since you're in charge of the decisions you make, you don't need to feel guilty if you consciously decided to eat more than necessary.

Instead, regret means you dislike how you feel and wish you hadn't eaten so much. It leaves the door open for you to learn from the experience so you can do a little better next time. Even people who eat instinctively overeat for convenience or pleasure. They sometimes regret it later, but since they don't feel guilty about it, it doesn't lead to more overeating and restrictive eating to make up for it.

Don't Miss the Lesson

When you realize your blood glucose is above target from overeating, ask yourself, *Why did it happen?* Some other questions to help you determine why you overate are:

- *Why did I eat in the first place? Was I in an instinctive, a restrictive, or an overeating cycle?*

- *When did I get the urge to eat? What was I thinking? What was I feeling? What else was happening?*

- *Can I identify hunger? Was I hungry? How hungry was I?*

- *If I wasn't hungry, what was the physical, emotional, or environmental trigger?*

- *What did I choose to eat and why? Did that affect how much I ate?*

- *How did I eat? Was I mindful or distracted?*

- *Did I set an intention for how full I wanted be afterward?*

- *How much food did I have in front of me?*

- *What was I thinking about when I decided to continue eating past the point of satisfaction?*

Most important, ask yourself, *What could I do differently next time?* Developing a strategy for what you'll do differently turns your mistake into a learning experience.

To help you sort it out, let's go back through the mindful eating cycle to explore possible triggers for overeating and strategies for dealing with them more effectively. This will be a great review and application of some of the concepts you discovered in previous chapters. Go back and reread any sections you're struggling with.

Why?

It just happened. When you don't decide ahead of time how you want to feel after the meal, you're more likely to overeat. In other words, start eating with an intention, such as, *I'll eat only as much as I need to feel comfortable at level 5.*

You can always change your mind, but don't let it just happen; decide with full awareness of the consequences.

I've been feeling deprived. If you've been in a restrictive eating cycle, you're more likely to overeat when you finally give in to cravings. Remind yourself that there are no good or bad foods. You're less likely to feel out of control around food when you know you can have it again whenever you want it.

I was rebelling. If someone said you can't or shouldn't eat something, you may eat more to spite that person. But ultimately, whom have you punished? Since you're the one in charge of your eating, you get to choose when, what, and how much you'll eat.

I always overeat in that situation. Many people learn to associate certain events with overeating: Thanksgiving dinner, sporting events, dinner at Grandmother's house. Be aware of these triggers so that you can think them through in advance and create new strategies that suit you better.

It was a special occasion. You're more likely to overeat if you give yourself permission to eat enjoyable foods only on special occasions. You don't need an excuse to have a wonderful meal. Why use a special occasion as a reason to overeat? Just ask yourself, *If this occasion is so special, why would I want to eat until I'm uncomfortable?*

I felt obligated. You may sometimes feel expected to eat, such as when someone else made or bought the food. Other people may urge you to eat for many reasons, for example, to make themselves feel good, to show you they care about you, or to avoid eating alone. Feeling obligated can cause you to ignore your body's signals of satisfaction to please someone else or as an excuse to overeat. Remember, you eat to meet your body's needs, so come up with some polite but firm responses in advance.

When?

I wasn't hungry when I started eating. When you eat before you're hungry, just about any amount of food will make you feel full. Ramona is working on freeing herself from eating on a schedule:

> *My husband has always been an instinctive eater. Sometimes I'd get so mad at him because I'd work all afternoon preparing lasagna or something else special for dinner, but some days he'd just pick at it. He'd say he*

just wasn't very hungry because they'd gone out for lunch. I used to try to get him to eat anyway, because I thought, Hey, it's lasagna, I made it, and you should want to eat it, no matter what else you ate today! *But now I understand and I've stopped pushing food on him.*

In fact, I realized that a lot of times, I wasn't really all that hungry at dinnertime either. It dawned on me that I taste a lot while I cook. I'm trying to break that habit, but now, if one of us isn't hungry, we just wrap it up to have for lunch or dinner the next day, when we'll actually enjoy it.

I was too hungry when I started eating. When you wait too long to eat, you're more likely to eat too much, too quickly, and therefore overshoot your stomach's comfortable capacity. Pay more attention to your hunger cues and be prepared to eat when you get to level 2 or 3. If you're at level 1, look closely for any signs and symptoms of hypoglycemia (see chapter 5). Test your blood glucose (if possible) and treat hypoglycemia appropriately. If your blood glucose is in the target range but you're very hungry, slow down, eat a little at first to allow your blood glucose to come up gradually, and stay mindful of your choices.

I might be overeating to stuff other feelings. This is the most challenging reason for eating beyond satisfaction. It may also be the most important. If you eat rather than feel your feelings or cope with your emotions, you can't meet your true needs. The first step is to become aware of what's happening; thereafter, make a decision to work on it, one step at a time.

What?

It tasted good, so I just kept eating. Your taste buds are the most sensitive when you're hungry and when you first start eating, so that's when food tastes the best. You might keep eating because you want to reexperience those first wonderful bites, but by then, you are really just eating a memory. It won't taste that wonderful until you're hungry again. When you're eating a delicious food, don't get so caught up in the experience that you don't notice how you actually feel or forget how you'll feel if you overeat. Check in and remind yourself that if you keep eating, the discomfort will eventually outweigh the enjoyment.

I wanted to taste everything. Having a lot of food to choose from causes people to eat more. If you know it's difficult for you to have a lot of choices, you may wish to avoid buffets and similar settings whenever possible. Better yet, turn it around. Decide that with so many choices, you'll get to eat exactly what you want. You can be extremely picky; decide that you will only eat what you love and won't bother with anything that's just so-so.

I was afraid I wouldn't get that food again. You may convince yourself that this is the only time you'll get to have a particular food so you should eat all you can. But it's rare that a food will never be available again. You can ask for the recipe, take some home, ask the cook to make it for you again sometime, plan to return to the same restaurant, or enjoy experimenting with similar foods in the future.

I saved the best for last. If you save your favorite food for the end of your meal, you might eat it even if you're already full (this applies to dessert too). Instead, have a bite or two when it will taste the best. Then, if you're too full to finish it, it will be easier to save the rest for later.

I ate food I didn't enjoy. Choosing food that isn't really what you want will probably leave you less satisfied. You may continue to eat, trying to reach satisfaction without realizing that the food choice, not the amount, is the problem. If you realize you're eating a food you don't really enjoy, stop and choose something else. If there are no other options, eat cautiously and promise yourself to eat something you like at the next meal.

How?

I wasn't paying attention as I ate. You can't pay full attention to two things simultaneously, so when you eat while doing something else, you're less likely to enjoy your food or notice when you've had enough. Instead, choose to savor each bite without other distractions.

I ate too fast. When you eat quickly, your brain may not realize your stomach is full until it's too late. Slow down and pause for at least two minutes in the middle of eating to reconnect and ask yourself where you are on the Hunger and Fullness Scale.

I mindlessly picked at leftovers. When you reach your intended level of fullness, get up from the table, clear the food or have someone remove your plate, and package up leftovers for another meal.

How Much?

I had too much on my plate. Generally, the larger the serving size, the more food you'll eat. Make it a point to serve yourself only as much as you think you'll need. When you've been given a larger portion than necessary, divide it into a more appropriate portion or, better yet, have the excess wrapped to go.

I was keeping up with someone else. You may overeat when someone else is eating a lot or eating very fast. You might be afraid you won't get your share or think you're not eating that much compared to the other person. Remember, you're eating for you, no one else.

I'm used to feeling full after a meal. Over time, you may have grown used to that full feeling from overeating. In the past, it may have even been your only signal to stop. If you're having difficulty letting that go, try drinking water when you eat, eating soup before your meal, and enjoying plenty of high-fiber fruits and vegetables and salads to fill you up without adding a lot more calories than your body needs. Also practice noticing all the negative consequences from being too full. Eventually, most people begin to view fullness as an unpleasant state they want to avoid.

I wanted to get my money's worth. Paying for a meal may tempt you to eat more than necessary to avoid feeling that you've wasted your money. You might also be tempted to buy (and then eat) more than necessary because it's a better value. Whenever you eat more than your body needs, your money is wasted anyway.

I hate to let food go to waste. This may come from your childhood: "Eat all your dinner; there are starving children in (fill in the blank)." Eating all your food doesn't help children anywhere. If you're concerned about wasting food, take smaller portions, share meals, and save leftovers to eat later.

I wanted to earn my dessert. You are an adult now; you don't have to clean your plate if you want dessert. Instead, update that other familiar phrase, "Save room for dessert!" to "Save a carbohydrate choice for dessert!"

Where?

I kept eating to avoid or postpone doing something else. Sometimes eating is a lot easier or more fun than whatever else you think you should do. To combat this problem, make sure you have something to look forward to (or at least that you don't dread) after eating.

I'd rather eat than do just about anything else. If you don't have other things you enjoy doing that make you feel good, you may eat for pleasure and to "fill" yourself up. See chapter 21 for other ways to nourish your body, mind, heart, and spirit.

If your underlying reasons for overeating still aren't apparent, they may be buried under denial or other coping mechanisms. If your overeating continues without any progress toward identifying and addressing your triggers, professional guidance will probably help.

Strategies: *I Ate Too Much! Now What?*

When you overeat, it's very helpful to let it go and reenter your instinctive eating cycle at your next decision point.

After eating, sit quietly for a few moments and become completely aware of how you feel and where your energy is going. When you've eaten too much, your stomach is distended, your blood glucose rises, and you may feel sluggish as your body processes and stores the excess fuel you consumed. Again, don't beat yourself up; just focus on the sensations so you can remember them in detail. That way, the next time you're tempted to overeat, you can recall how you felt when you were overfull, and you'll be less likely to repeat that mistake.

Why? People who eat instinctively sometimes overeat. Although they probably feel regretful and uncomfortable, they don't typically feel guilty. Therefore, they don't think, *Well, I've already blown it; I might as well keep eating and start my diet tomorrow.* Those thoughts would only trap them in an eat-repent-repeat cycle. Instead, they just listen to their bodies and return to eating instinctively by allowing hunger to drive the next cycle.

When? When you've overeaten, wait to see when you get hungry again. Rather than continue eating out of guilt or because it's time, listen to your body. It probably won't need food again as soon; therefore, you may not be hungry for your usual snack or even your next meal.

What? Don't penalize yourself or try to compensate for overeating by restricting yourself. If you try to make yourself eat foods you don't really want, you'll feel deprived and punished, fueling your eat-repent-repeat cycle. When you get hungry again, ask yourself, *What do I want?* and *What do I need?* Trust and respect the wisdom of your body, which will probably naturally seek balance, variety, and moderation. You might notice that you're hungry for something small or light: maybe a bowl of soup or cereal, a piece of fruit, or a salad.

How? Eating mindfully with intention and attention will help you to be less likely to repeat your recent mistake.

How much? You may not be as hungry, so pay close attention to how much you serve, order, prepare, and eat.

Where? Don't use exercise to punish yourself for overeating; instead, be active and use your fuel to live a full and satisfying life!

Here's how Janette addressed one of her triggers for overeating:

I was doing really well. I wasn't overeating like I used to, and my diabetes was under control. Then I started dealing with problems at both home and work. I felt frustrated and overwhelmed all the time, and I wasn't sleeping well. I started eating more, and my blood sugar climbed. At first, I started telling myself I can't have this, and I can't have that, which just made me want it more. I started to feel afraid, because it felt like I was dieting again. It took me a while to realize that I had slipped back into my old restrictive eating cycle. That had never worked for very long, so I renewed my commitment to eat mindfully. I really focused on using the Hunger and Fullness Scale to guide my eating. I saw my blood sugar improve right away. I also became more aware of my impulses to eat to soothe stress. I felt better and had more energy to deal with my problems, and everything seemed to settle back down.

With practice, you'll prefer feeling contented and comfortable after eating. When you feel too full or your blood glucose spikes after eating, try to figure out why, and develop a plan for what to do differently next time. Perfection isn't possible or even necessary, so just get right back into your instinctive eating cycle by waiting to see when you get hungry again and what you're hungry for. With practice, it becomes easier and more natural to stop eating when you feel just right.

CHAPTER 18

Care:
Problem Solving

There are a number of challenges that most people with diabetes have to deal with at one time or another. The following list of common issues may improve your understanding of how to identify problems, find possible solutions, and take appropriate action:

- Staying motivated to monitor your glucose

- Handling blood glucose problems (lows and highs)

- Managing a missed medication dose

- Coping with injury or illness

Respond instead of React

Problems can be inconvenient, uncomfortable, or even scary. These feelings are natural, but how you *respond* determines how much of an effect they'll have and how long it will take to get back on track. Notice that we intentionally chose the word "respond" instead of "react." This is an important distinction when you remember that your thoughts and feelings are closely linked to your actions and results, as we discussed in chapter 4 (see figure 4.1).

Reactions are based on past experiences and established beliefs, which trigger familiar thoughts and feelings. Therefore, when you react, you repeat previous actions based on what happened in the past. Not surprisingly, when you react, you probably get the same results as in the past. Sometimes reacting can be helpful, for example, when you react rapidly to treat low blood glucose by taking the appropriate actions you've learned from prior experiences. On the other hand, when you replay ineffective thoughts, feelings, and actions you will probably get undesirable results again and again. Even a lack of action, when action is needed is an ineffective reaction.

You may not be aware of what you're thinking, feeling, or doing until you're faced with one of these problems. Being mindful teaches you to pause and notice your thoughts and feelings without judgment so you can decide whether they are really helping you in the current situation. With that awareness, you can choose to respond to what's happening now. This allows you to thoughtfully consider your options and choose the actions that will bring you the results you want rather than re-create the past again and again. When you respond, you take responsibility for choosing your actions.

Strategies: How Would You Respond?

Recall times when you've faced the following situations. If they haven't come up yet, imagine what you'd do. Take a piece of paper and spend a few minutes writing down your honest answers to the following questions for each situation:

What do you think?

How do you feel?

What would you do?

What would happen?

Situation 1: You have a follow-up appointment with your doctor in a few days but have only checked your blood glucose a few times since your last visit.

Situation 2: You're shopping at the mall with a friend when you start feeling light-headed, sweaty, and a little shaky.

Situation 3: Your blood glucose has been above target for the last two days.

Situation 4: You are at a ball game, when you remember that you forgot to take your diabetes medication.

Situation 5: You caught a bad cold and have lost your appetite.

As we explore problem-solving skills related to situations you'll probably face when you have diabetes, see if you'd make any changes in the way you think and feel about—and respond to—these situations in the future.

Staying Motivated to Monitor Your Blood Glucose

If you're like most people, there will be times and situations when you simply don't want to check your blood glucose. There are many reasons for this; perhaps you feel that it's not worth the effort, time, or cost. Maybe there are times when you question the helpfulness of the information or even the accuracy of your meter. Sometimes resistance stems from underlying feelings about having diabetes. Staying motivated to monitor your blood glucose levels begins with recognizing that it's normal to feel this way at times.

Are Your Thoughts on Your Side?

We initially explored examples of ineffective and effective thoughts in chapter 4. Let's examine how two of those thought patterns affect your ability to motivate yourself to monitor your blood glucose.

Self-Defeating vs. Affirming

I don't have the energy (or *time* or *money*) *to check my blood glucose all the time* is a self-defeating thought. Ironically, high blood glucose leaves you feeling fatigued, sleepy, and less energetic, while low blood glucose can leave you feeling drained physically, mentally, and emotionally. Sometimes people associate these feelings with monitoring when the feelings are actually due to high or low blood glucose—which you can only manage when you're aware of it.

A more-affirming thought is, *When I know my blood glucose, I'm in charge of my diabetes instead of letting high or low blood glucose hijack my life.* Think of monitoring your blood glucose as an investment in your health. Acknowledge that there will be days when you're tempted to spend your energy, time, or money on something other than focusing on your goal of optimal glucose management. Remind yourself that monitoring requires less energy, time, and money than dealing with the consequences of not knowing until problems arise. Fortunately, as blood glucose technology continues to advance, testing is quicker, more affordable, and less uncomfortable than before.

Negative vs. Positive

I know I should monitor, but I hate it when the numbers are high. Such negative thoughts and feelings can stem from resistance to being told what to do; frustration about the inconvenience, discomfort, or cost of testing; ambivalence about taking action based on the numbers; and anger that people around you don't appreciate your effort to manage your diabetes. As a result, monitoring feels like a chore instead of a tool, making it less likely that you'll test and, therefore, causing you to miss an opportunity to address problems. As a result, the numbers are more likely to be high, thus reinforcing the initial negative thoughts.

Knowing my blood glucose gives me information that helps me take steps to care for my diabetes is a more positive thought. When you approach testing with curiosity rather than resistance, you'll see the numbers as information rather than judgment. The results can affirm the changes and choices you've made or encourage you to make further adjustments. Choosing to start monitoring your blood glucose this week will increase your understanding of your diabetes and create many small but powerful opportunities to improve your health.

If you find yourself having difficulty staying motivated to check your blood glucose regularly, explore the underlying thoughts and feelings as well as new, more effective thoughts.

Problems with Your Blood Glucose

The goal of blood glucose management is to keep your blood glucose levels in the target range that prevents complications and helps you feel your best. Both low and high blood glucose can disrupt your life and lead to serious short- and long-term consequences. Therefore, it's important to know how to identify blood glucose problems, respond appropriately, and take action to prevent them in the future.

Hypoglycemia (Low Blood Glucose)

Hypoglycemia is defined as a blood glucose level of less than 70 mg/dL. Having diabetes does not cause hypoglycemia, but some of the medications you may need to take to lower your blood glucose can potentially cause it to drop too low. Ask your health care provider if any of your medications can cause hypoglycemia. If you are at risk for hypoglycemia, carry glucose tablets or gel with you, wear a medical bracelet, and be sure that others you spend time with are aware of emergency instructions too.

Hypoglycemia is usually mild and can be treated quickly and easily by eating or drinking a small amount of glucose-rich food (see below). The symptoms of hypoglycemia include hunger, shakiness, nervousness, sweating, dizziness or light-headedness, sleepiness, confusion, difficulty speaking, anxiety, and weakness. If left untreated, hypoglycemia can get worse and cause confusion, clumsiness, or fainting. Severe hypoglycemia can lead to seizures, coma, and even death.

In addition to the immediate problems hypoglycemia causes, having repeated low blood-glucose reactions over time can lead to a condition called *hypoglycemia unawareness*, which, just as the name of this condition indicates, is the inability to recognize low blood glucose. As a result, blood glucose can fall dangerously low, leading to weakness, confusion, or unconsciousness, preventing you from treating the low blood glucose by yourself.

This section will review the treatment of hypoglycemia and help you uncover what caused an episode of low blood glucose so that you can take steps to prevent it in the future.

What to Do When Your Blood Glucose Is Low

Before low blood glucose occurs, be sure that you (and people you spend time with) understand how to treat it and that you are prepared at all times.

Test. If you have symptoms of hypoglycemia, test your blood glucose if possible. If it's impossible to test, then treat it anyway.

Treat. If your blood glucose is less than 70 mg/dL (or you can't test), treat your low blood glucose with 15 to 20 grams of carbohydrate. Examples include an appropriate dose of glucose tablets or gel, four ounces of juice or soda (not diet), six saltine crackers, four to five pieces of roll candy (such as Life Savers), one tablespoon of sugar or honey, or whatever your health care provider advises. If you are unable to consume carbohydrate by mouth, 911 should be called immediately.

Retest and re-treat if needed. Wait fifteen minutes and retest. If your blood glucose remains low, re-treat with 15 grams of carbohydrates. These steps should be repeated until the blood glucose level is 70 mg/dL or above. If your next meal is an hour or more away, eat a snack such as half a sandwich, yogurt, or peanut butter and crackers.

Track. Keep a careful log of all your low blood-glucose readings to look for patterns and identify possible causes and solutions. For example, does it happen at a particular time of day or after a certain type of activity?

Follow up. If you have two or more low blood-glucose readings in a week, call your health care provider. Based on your log, you might be asked to add snacks or adjust what, when, and how much medication you take.

Identifying the Causes of Low Blood Glucose

You can usually trace the causes of low blood glucose back to changes in eating, physical activity, or medications. Occasionally, the cause isn't obvious, so you'll need to do a little more digging.

Changes in eating. Missing or delaying a meal, eating different food, or eating less food can all lead to hypoglycemia. When you have low blood glucose, review your most recent eating cycle to see if the cause was when, what, or how much you ate. Barbara shares what happened when there was a sudden change in what she ate:

> My coworker invited my husband and me over to his home a few weeks ago to eat dinner and play cards. Right before the meal, his wife said they were on a low-carb diet and proudly announced that we wouldn't be having any bread, pasta, starchy vegetables, or dessert with the meal. I had already taken my usual medications but was too embarrassed to say anything about my diabetes. I tried eating extra vegetables and meat but knew they didn't contain many carbohydrates. We played cards for a couple of hours after dinner, and then my husband started teasing me about the stupid hands I was playing. I decided I'd better check my blood sugar, and, sure enough, it was 68. I took four glucose tabs from my purse and explained what was happening. I guess I embarrassed myself anyway, but at least I learned my lesson! I know that changes in my diet can affect my blood glucose, so I'll ask what's for dinner ahead of time.

Running late, having a busy day, or dealing with other unexpected interruptions can affect when, what, and how much you eat. Planning, preparation, and anticipation can help you deal with these situations. If you're at risk for hypoglycemia, carry glucose tabs or gel, or another source of glucose with you at all times. If you continue to experience low blood glucose, talk to your health care professional about changing your medications. If a medication change isn't appropriate, work with a dietitian to plan your snacks and meals to coordinate with the peak onset of action of your glucose-lowering medications.

More exercise than usual. As you learned in chapters 8 and 12, exercise is a very effective way to lower your blood glucose. When you exercise more than you anticipated, your blood glucose can drop too low. Stephen learned this the hard way:

> *My wife and I celebrated our twenty-fifth wedding anniversary in France. People walk everywhere there, so we did too. One afternoon we got lost on our way to lunch. We walked around in circles for over half an hour. By the time we got to the restaurant, I was trembling and starting to feel clammy. I had taken my usual medications that morning, so I suspected that with all that extra exercise, I was probably having a low blood sugar reaction. I didn't have my meter with me, but I ate a piece of French bread as soon as we sat down and felt better within ten minutes.*

Too much medication. The type of medication and dosage are determined by your lab results (such as A1C), blood glucose log, other medical conditions, and lifestyle (including eating and physical activity patterns). As your diet and activity improve, you often need less medication. This is good news—as long as you and your health care team make the necessary adjustments. Laura provides a good example of this situation:

> *I've had diabetes for over ten years. I tried and tried but just couldn't stick to a meal plan or regular exercise. My blood sugar levels were often above target, even though I was on three medications. When I learned about mindful eating, it just clicked! I was making healthier choices, and I even got a dog and started walking him twice a day. I was actually excited about my next diabetes checkup because I wanted to show my doctor my blood sugar log. Turns out, I couldn't wait that long: I had three low blood sugars in a row, so I called and they got me right in. She was really happy with all the changes I'd made but reminded me that she needs to make adjustments to my medications whenever there's a significant change in my eating or exercise.*

Hyperglycemia (High Blood Glucose)

Your health care provider will establish a target range for your blood glucose. As you know, elevated blood-glucose levels increase your risk for kidney disease, retinopathy, and neuropathy, and they play a role in heart disease, delayed healing, and infection. They can also cause you to feel fatigued.

Identifying the Causes of High Blood Glucose

The causes of high blood glucose can often be traced back to changes in eating, physical activity, and medication. In addition, an injury, illness, infection, or stress can cause a sudden increase in blood glucose. More gradual changes may be from increasing insulin resistance, decreasing insulin production, and age-related changes.

Changes in eating. When your blood glucose is too high, the mindful eating cycle provides clues to possible causes, as you learned in "Don't Miss the Lesson" in chapter 17.

Overtreatment of hypoglycemia. Hypoglycemia can be an unpleasant experience, so you might be tempted to overtreat it by eating until you feel better. But overeating doesn't raise your blood glucose *faster* than eating 15 grams of carbohydrate or taking four glucose tabs, and it can raise your blood glucose *higher* than it needs to go.

Changes in physical activity. Less physical activity than normal can lead to a higher blood glucose than normal, as Jason discovered:

> My blood glucose was high when I woke up this morning. I reviewed my eating from yesterday, but nothing was out of the ordinary. Then I remembered that I'd skipped my walk after work because it was raining. I looked through my blood glucose log and realized what a difference exercise makes.

Changes in medication. Another possible cause of high blood glucose to consider is a missed dose or other changes to your medication.

Illness. Having a cold or flu is a stress on the body that can cause blood glucose to rise. Additionally, being sick can change activity and eating patterns.

Medication side effects. Some over-the-counter and prescribed medications are known to raise your blood glucose, including cough syrup, certain antidepressants, inhalers, steroids (such as those taken for a flare-up of asthma or injections in your joints), and others. Make sure that all of your health care providers (including your pharmacist) are aware that you have diabetes.

Progression of diabetes. Diabetes is not a static disease; in other words, you can expect it to change over time. Learn from Luke's experience:

> My blood glucose had been in the target range most of the time for over a year. It started to creep up gradually for no apparent reason. The changes were pretty small, but it was getting higher and higher. I guess I was just waiting to see what would happen. I was surprised when my doctor told me my A1C had gone up two points, but I guess I shouldn't have been. I'll pay more attention to small changes before they add up to big ones.

What to Do When Your Blood Glucose Is High

It's important to talk to your health care provider about what to do when your blood glucose is high since specific instructions will vary by your type of diabetes (type 1 or 2), how high your blood glucose is, and other factors, like your age and medical condition. The following are general guidelines.

Blood glucose over target but less than 250 mg/dL. If you have type 2 diabetes, a blood glucose level above target but less than 250 mg/dL is best treated by increased fluid intake and gentle activity. Good options for fluids include water, herbal tea, or zero-calorie, decaffeinated beverages. Examples of gentle activity include walking, light yard work, light housework, and gentle yoga. Recheck your glucose before your next meal or at bedtime, whichever comes first, to make sure it's coming down.

If you notice that your blood glucose level has been elevated for more than a week without changes to your diet, activity, or overall health, make an appointment with your doctor.

Blood glucose over 250 mg/dL. Discuss with your doctor what steps to take when your blood glucose is over 250 mg/dL. If you are taking insulin, you will be instructed about any necessary adjustments to your insulin dose. (If you have type 1 diabetes, you may also be asked to check your blood or urine for ketones.) If your blood glucose remains elevated despite taking the recommended insulin dose, contact your doctor. You may need emergency medical treatment for intravenous hydration and insulin management.

Managing a Missed Medication Dose

Nobody's perfect! We all have off days, make a mistake, or find ourselves unsure of what to do. Since there are many different types of medications for diabetes, each of which works differently (as we described in chapter 10), there's no rule of thumb about what to do for missed doses. When you start a new medication, ask your health care professional what to do if you miss a dose.

If you find that you're missing doses of medication regularly, figure out why. Is it because the instructions are confusing or the dosing regimen is too complicated? Are you feeling distracted or overwhelmed? Are you having difficulty affording your medications? Work with your health care professional to explore solutions and options. Here's what Vickie found:

I kept missing my lunchtime insulin dose and making excuses about why. I finally had to have a gentle heart-to-heart talk with myself. I realized that I didn't like checking my blood glucose or injecting insulin in front of others, especially my coworkers, because I didn't want them to feel uncomfortable. I decided to stop putting myself at risk and began planning my workday better so I would have some privacy before lunch. Thinking about what I need to do to care for myself put me back in charge.

Coping with an Illness or Injury

Illness and injury cause the release of various hormones (cortisol, epinephrine, growth hormone, and glucagon) that can lead to increased blood glucose. High blood glucose can prolong the course of an illness and delay healing, resulting in a vicious cycle. In addition, high blood glucose causes a loss of fluid (remember that you have polyuria when your glucose is high). This, along with fever, vomiting, or diarrhea, can lead to dehydration, requiring immediate medical attention. With type 1 diabetes, if the high blood glucose isn't treated with enough insulin, a life-threatening condition called *diabetic ketoacidosis* (DKA) can develop.

To prevent serious complications, such as dehydration, DKA, or delayed healing, it's important to recognize illnesses and injuries early and to treat the illness *and* high blood glucose appropriately. In addition, prolonged illness or injury, or recovery from surgery will require adjustments to your diabetes treatment to support healing.

Prevention Is the Best Medicine, of Course!

It's always best to prevent illness and injury whenever possible. We discussed some of the preventive measures you can take, like getting vaccinated against influenza and pneumonia and taking good care of your feet. Review chapter 14 for other steps you can take to keep yourself as healthy as possible.

Sick-Day Guidelines

The primary goal of establishing and following sick-day guidelines is to prevent dehydration and keep your blood glucose under control.

Monitor your blood glucose closely. Test your blood glucose more often to be sure that it isn't going too high or too low.

Drink plenty of fluids. Remember, high blood glucose causes an excessive loss of fluid because the body is pulling fluid from the cells to dilute the concentrated blood glucose. In addition, fever, vomiting, and diarrhea can also lead to dehydration. Try to drink eight to ten ounces of water every hour to prevent dehydration.

Continue to take your medications. The stress of being sick causes your blood glucose to rise, so continue to take your medications even when you're sick. However, if you can't eat solid food due to nausea, vomiting, or diarrhea, there's an increased risk of developing low blood glucose. Therefore sip beverages that contain carbohydrate, such as ginger ale, sports drinks, or juice, or consume flavored gelatin or ice pops (not the sugar-free kind).

Seek immediate medical attention if your illness is severe. If you develop the following symptoms, call your doctor or go to the emergency room:

- Vomiting more than once

- Diarrhea more than five times in less than twenty-four hours

- Inability to take fluids by mouth

- Becoming weaker

- Difficulty breathing or rapid and labored respirations

- Moderate or large ketones that do not improve after twelve to twenty-four hours following treatment (if type 1)

- Change in mental status, such as confusion or loss of consciousness

- Blood glucose over 250 mg/dL on two consecutive checks despite increased insulin dose (as recommended by your health care professional)

As you can appreciate after this review of common problems, diabetes is not a static condition. Therefore, it's impossible to put it on autopilot and move on. However, with consistent self-care, awareness, and responsiveness, it *is* possible to attain optimal health with diabetes.

CHAPTER 19

Nourish:
Protein Power

F ound in every cell in your body, protein plays a role in basic bodily functions, ranging from walking to digesting food. It's critical for building
muscle and vital for optimal health. Eating protein also promotes the
greatest satiety of the three macronutrients (Gerstein et al. 2004). The satiety
that comes from eating protein made a big difference for Leigh Ann:

> As I became aware of when, what, and how much I was eating, I saw a
> strong connection between what I ate and my hunger levels. For example,
> I liked to eat an apple for my afternoon snack, but it never seemed to fill
> me up, so I would have another snack a short time later. When I tried
> putting a little peanut butter on my apple, I had enough energy to make it
> the rest of the afternoon, and my blood sugars were more in my target
> range. Now I keep nuts, string cheese, slices of turkey, and other high-
> protein snacks on hand so I'm not running back to the kitchen all
> afternoon.

Why Is Protein Important?

- It increases satiety so that you feel fuller, longer.

- It builds, repairs, and maintains healthy muscles, organs, skin,
  and hair.

- It manufactures enzymes and hormones, blood-clotting factors.

- It maintains water balance, transports oxygen, regulates acid-base balance, and supports immune function.

- It provides the body with four calories of energy per gram.

- It contributes essential nutrients; for example, dairy products are a significant source of calcium, and beef is an excellent source of iron. Dairy products and meat also provide zinc, as well as vitamins B_6 and B_{12}.

What Is Protein Anyway?

Protein is made up of nitrogen-containing building blocks called *amino acids*. During digestion, proteins is broken down to provide amino acids and nitrogen for your body. Just as the letters of the alphabet are arranged in different ways to make words, the twenty amino acids are arranged in different ways to build proteins with specific forms and functions.

Amino acids are classified as essential and nonessential. They're all important, but you must eat the nine essential amino acids because your body cannot manufacture them. Your body can manufacture the other eleven nonessential amino acids with the nitrogen it gets from any amino acid.

Animal protein sources, such as meat, poultry, fish, eggs, and dairy products, and plant sources, such as soybeans and quinoa, contain all of the essential amino acids. Other plant sources, including grains, beans, lentils, nuts, and seeds, contain various essential amino acids. By eating a variety of these foods, you can consume all of the amino acids necessary to make the proteins your body needs.

How Much Do I Need?

Based on recommendations from various authorities, your protein intake should fall in the range of 10 to 35 percent of your total calories per day. On average, healthy women between the ages of nineteen and seventy need approximately 46 grams of protein a day; healthy men in this age range need approximately 56 grams of protein a day to avoid deficiency. In general, healthy adults should consume 0.8 to 1.2 grams of protein for every kilogram of lean body weight (1 kilogram equals 2.2 pounds).

A woman could easily consume 46 grams of protein by drinking an 8-ounce glass of low-fat milk in the morning, eating a sandwich made with a 3-ounce chicken breast for lunch, having 1 ounce of nuts as a snack, and eating half a cup of beans at dinnertime. A man could add 3 ounces of beef or fish to dinner to meet his protein requirements. Of course, these examples don't include the proteins in grains, vegetables, or additional dairy products, which would further increase their intake. The point is that you can easily meet your daily protein needs without consuming a large amount of food.

Protein

Typical Serving Sizes

Beef, Pork, Poultry, Fish .... 3–4 ounces (palm-sized)

Cheese .... 1 ounce or 1 slice

Cottage cheese .... 1/2 cup

Deli meat .... 2–3 ounces, 4–6 thin slices

Egg .... 1 large

Egg whites .... 2 large

Tofu .... 4 ounces or 1/2 cup

Figure 19.1

Strategies: How Do You Optimize Your Intake of Protein?

The following strategies will help you make healthy protein choices.

Be selective. Protein from animal sources may contain a significant amount of saturated fat, cholesterol, or both (see chapter 15). Select round and loin cuts of beef and pork. Select the leanest available ground beef. Use skinless chicken or turkey breast. When possible, select low-fat or fat-free dairy products, such as skim or 1 percent milk, buttermilk, cottage cheese with 2 percent or less fat, low-fat yogurt, and low-fat cheeses. When lean or lower-fat versions don't make the cut for your taste preferences and you opt for higher-fat versions instead, be selective about how often you consume them and how much you eat.

Eat more fish. Fatty fish is high in omega-3 fatty acids and protein. Aim for two 4-ounce servings of fish each week.

Experiment with plant-based proteins. Plant-based proteins, like beans, legumes, whole grains, quinoa, and nuts, are typically fiber and nutrient rich, and naturally low in saturated fat and cholesterol. Some plant sources of protein, like nuts, are also high in polyunsaturated fat. Going meatless sometimes is a healthful move because it has been shown to reduce the risk of heart disease, stroke, obesity, some forms of cancer, and adult-onset diabetes. It can be as easy as choosing meatless chili, vegetarian stir-fry, or salad topped with nuts or low-fat beans. Or you can be more adventurous, incorporating exotic grains, tofu, and ethnic vegetarian specialties. You may even want to designate certain meatless meals or days like "Meatless Monday." Striking the right balance depends on your taste preferences and lifestyle.

Preparation is important. Choose items that are grilled, broiled, baked, or poached instead of fried or served with heavy butter- or cream-based sauces. For flavor, marinate meats, poultry, and fish in low-fat dressings, sprinkle with a special seasoning mixture, or rub with a flavorful blend of herbs and spices.

Balance, Variety, and Moderation

How will you practice balance, variety, and moderation? Balance your intake of other macronutrients with protein, which helps you feel satisfied sooner and longer. Consume protein from a variety of animal and plant sources for optimal nutrients; for example, red meat is high in iron, fish is high in omega-3 fatty acids, dairy is high in calcium, legumes are high in fiber, and nuts are high in beneficial unsaturated fats. Practice moderation; limit animal sources of protein that are high in saturated fat and cholesterol.

CHAPTER 20

Live:
Increase Your Flexibility

S tretching feels good. Animals, including humans, stretch instinctively. You've probably seen dogs or cats stretch spontaneously, almost lazily, naturally tuning up all their muscles. Infants will arch their backs and stretch their arms when you pick them up after a nap. After sitting in one position too long, you naturally stretch to relieve stiffness. If this spontaneous stretching can feel that good, imagine how good it will feel to stretch all your muscles regularly as part of your overall fitness program.

Why Bother?

Flexibility is a key part of a complete and balanced fitness program. Flexibility is the ability of your joints to move through their full range of motion. Stretching exercises increase your flexibility through gentle stretching movements that increase the length of your muscles and connective tissues around your joints. Francine gives us a great example of why this is so important:

> I swear, all I was doing was wrapping Christmas presents. I reached for some ribbon and strained my back. How do you explain that to your friends without feeling ridiculous?

As Francine learned the hard way, the many benefits of flexibility are as follows:

- It optimizes your ability to function in daily life.

- It enhances physical and mental relaxation by decreasing tension and stiffness in your muscles.

- It maintains and increases the range of motion in your joints by increasing the length of your muscles and tendons.

- It offsets age-related stiffness and may slow the degeneration of the joints.

- It helps you develop body awareness and improved coordination.

- It improves your posture and muscular balance. Stretching the muscles of the lower back, shoulders, and chest will help keep your back in better alignment and improve your posture.

- It decreases your risk of lower-back pain. Improved flexibility in the hamstrings, hip flexors, quadriceps, and other muscles attached to the pelvis will relieve tension on the lumbar spine and reduce the risk of lower-back pain.

- It makes you feel good.

What You Need to Know

Everybody benefits from stretching. The methods are gentle and easy, and they apply regardless of your age, natural flexibility, or fitness level. You don't have to get in shape to stretch, but even athletes rely on flexibility training for peak performance.

The best time to stretch is when your muscles are warm. Like taffy, a warm muscle is more elastic and relaxes more easily. Overstretching a cold muscle can cause injury. Therefore, if you plan to stretch before exercising, warm up first by walking or doing your scheduled cardiorespiratory activity at a light intensity for five to ten minutes. This will increase the elasticity of and circulation to the muscles. Remember, stretching is not the same as warming up.

Before exercise. When you stretch before working out (but after warming up, of course), gently stretch all the muscles you'll use. For example, if you plan to ride a bike, lightly stretch the muscles in the front and back of your thighs and lower legs.

During exercise. Take a moment to stretch during cardiorespiratory activities when you stop to rest or take a drink. While strength training, you can stretch the muscles you're using between each set.

After exercise. An important time to stretch is after you exercise. This will lengthen your muscles again and release the tightness that exercise may produce. Be sure to stretch all the muscles you used during your workout.

Any time. You can do gentle stretching any time you feel like it: in the morning to begin your day, while sitting in a car, at your desk, after a warm bath or shower, or while relaxing. Stretching is beneficial whenever you feel muscular stiffness or need to release nervous tension. A few minutes a day of gentle stretching can relax your body and mind.

Getting Started

It's important to listen to your body; you shouldn't experience any pain. Stretching should be peaceful, relaxing, and noncompetitive. Here are the basics of stretching. Of course, consult your doctor before starting any exercise program. Stretching feels good when done correctly.

Warm up. Make sure your muscles are warm before stretching; for example, walk at a comfortable pace for five to ten minutes.

Breathe. Exhale as you begin the stretch. Continue to take slow, rhythmical breaths throughout the stretch. Don't hold your breath.

Listen to your body. Start by slowly stretching to the point of mild, comfortable tension. Do not stretch to the point of pain.

Relax. Relax as you hold the stretch. The feeling of tension should subside as you hold the position. If it doesn't, ease off slightly and find a degree of tension that's comfortable. As you inhale, release the stretch slightly; as you exhale, relax farther into the stretch.

Hold. Hold the stretch for ten to thirty seconds. As you feel the tension decrease, you can increase the stretch until you feel a slight pull again.

Don't bounce! Bouncing activates the stretch reflex that causes tightening of the muscles; it is counterproductive and can cause injury.

Repeat. When time allows, repeat each stretch two or three times for optimal benefit.

Fitness Rx: FITT Formula for More Flexibility

Remember to use the four points of the FITT Formula when working toward becoming more flexible.

- *Frequency:* Plan to stretch at least two to three times per week.

- *Intensity:* Gently stretch to the point of comfortable tension.

- *Time:* At first, hold each stretch for ten seconds; gradually increase the duration to thirty seconds. For optimal benefit, repeat each stretch three or four times.

- *Type:* Stretch specific muscle groups after exercise; try a stretch class, yoga, or Pilates.

Simple Stretches

Use the following flexibility exercises to stretch the specific muscle you used during a cardiorespiratory or strength-training session. For example, after a walk, cycling, or a lower-body strength-training session, do the lower-back and lower-leg stretches. After swimming, tennis, or upper-body strength training, do arm, chest, and upper-back stretches. Doing the entire sequence will allow these flexibility exercises to provide a good head-to-toe stretching session.

Neck Stretch

Muscles: Neck and upper back (trapezius)

1. Relax your neck muscles, bend your head, and bring your chin toward your chest. Hold for ten to thirty seconds.

2. Lift your chin and look up; hold.

3. Bring your head back to neutral and turn your head to one side, as though you were looking over your shoulder. Repeat on the opposite side.

4. Return your head to center and slowly lean your head to one side, bringing your ear toward your shoulder. You can place one hand on the side of your head to gently stretch the neck muscles farther. Repeat on the opposite side.

Shoulder Stretch

Muscles: Shoulders and upper back

1. Reach your right arm out in front of your body.

2. Place your left wrist on your right elbow and pull your right arm across your chest.

3. Keeping your right arm extended, use your left wrist to gently pull your right arm as close to your body as possible.

4. Relax your shoulders down, away from your ears. Hold for ten to thirty seconds. Repeat on the opposite side.

Triceps Stretch

Muscles: The triceps (located on the back of your upper arm) and shoulders

1. Raise your right arm toward the ceiling, and then bend your elbow and touch your neck or upper back with the palm of your right hand so that your right elbow points to the ceiling.

2. Grasp your right elbow with your left hand and pull it gently to the left until you feel a stretching sensation at the back of your upper right arm. Hold for ten to thirty seconds. Repeat on the opposite side.

Cat Stretch

Muscles: The entire back, including the cervical, thoracic, and lumbar vertebrae

1. Position yourself comfortably on your hands and knees, with your back level.

2. Inhale as you lift your head and tail and allow your back to sag.

3. Slowly exhale as you contract your stomach muscles and curve your back toward the ceiling, allowing your head to drop down and your tail to curve in. Hold for ten to thirty seconds.

4. Inhale as you slowly return to starting position. Exhale and then repeat.

Lower-Back Extension Stretch

Muscles: The abdominal and supporting muscles of the lower back (lumbar vertebrae)

1. Lie on your stomach and rest on your forearms, with your elbows positioned under your shoulders.

2. Gently raise your head and chest off the floor and look straight ahead, leaning comfortably on your forearms. You should feel a gentle stretch in your lower back and along the front of your body. Hold for ten to thirty seconds. Repeat.

Lower-Back Flexion Stretch

Muscles: The supporting muscles of the lower back (lumbar vertebrae)

1. Lie on your back, with both legs extended straight out.

2. Bend your right knee, clasp it with both hands, and then slowly pull the knee toward your chest. Hold for ten to thirty seconds.

3. Switch legs. Alternatively, you can pull both knees in at the same time.

Spinal Twist

Muscles: The entire back and the sides of your trunk

1. While seated on the floor, extend your right leg in front of you.

2. Bend your left leg and place your left foot on the outside of your right knee.

3. Extend your left arm behind you and place your left palm on the floor to support your body.

4. Use your right arm to gently twist your torso to the left until you feel the stretch along your right side and back. Hold for ten to thirty seconds. Repeat on the opposite side.

Inner-Thigh Stretch

Muscles: The inner thigh and groin muscles

1. While seated, pull both feet in toward your body with the soles facing each other.

2. Grasp your feet with your hands and press down slightly on your knees with your elbows. Hold for ten to thirty seconds.

Hamstring Stretch

Muscles: The hamstrings, located in the back of the upper legs

Sitting

1. Sit comfortably on the floor with your right leg straight and your left leg bent so that the sole of your left foot rests flat against the inside of your right leg.

2. While keeping your lower back straight, slowly reach toward your right foot until you feel a gentle stretching sensation in your right hamstring. During this stretch, keep your right foot pointing upward. Hold for ten to thirty seconds. Repeat on the opposite side.

Standing

1. Place your right foot about twelve inches in front of your left foot.

2. Lift the ball of your right foot and keep your leg straight.

3. Bend your back leg and lean forward into your front leg. Place your hands on your left thigh for balance. Hold for ten to thirty seconds. Repeat on the opposite side.

Chest Stretch

Muscles: Chest, shoulders, and back

1. Lace your fingers behind your back so that your palms face in toward your spine, thumbs pointing down at the ground.

2. Hold your chin up and lift your chest as high as you can.

3. Pull your shoulders back and lower your linked hands slightly toward the ground. Hold for ten to thirty seconds.

4. Release the tension and relax for a few seconds.

5. Now slowly raise your linked hands toward the ceiling, keeping your neck and back relaxed until you feel a gentle stretch in the front of your chest and shoulders.

Calf Stretch

Muscles: Calf muscles, located at the back of the lower leg

1. While standing, place your hands or forearms on a wall.

2. Place your right foot near the wall and, keeping your left foot flat on the floor, move your left leg back until you feel the stretch in the left calf muscle and the back of your ankle (Achilles tendon). Hold for ten to thirty seconds. Repeat on the opposite side.

Quadriceps Stretch

Muscles: Quadriceps (quads), located in the front of the thighs

1. Stand tall and support your body with your right hand against a wall or solid object for balance.

2. Raise your right heel toward your buttocks and then grasp your toes or ankle with your left hand.

3. Gently pull your heel up to your buttocks until you feel the stretch in your thigh. Hold for ten to thirty seconds. Repeat on the opposite side.

Modification: If you can't reach your toes or ankle, pull on your pant leg to raise your foot. Alternatively, you can rest your ankle on the seat of a chair placed behind you if that's enough of a stretch for the front of your thigh.

Stretch Your Limits: Yoga

Some people think yoga is just for flexible people, but, actually, it's a great form of exercise for everyone—particularly people who need to increase their flexibility! Yoga is a wonderful way to improve your flexibility, and it will improve your strength, stamina, and mindfulness too. People of all ages and levels of fitness can benefit from practicing yoga. Many of the stretches listed in the previous section are actually yoga postures.

Numerous styles of yoga and classes are available for all levels. Look for level 1, introductory, gentle, or beginners' DVDs or classes if you're new to yoga. If you don't like a particular class, try a different one. A yoga mat is essential because it provides a nonslip surface to keep you steady as you move in and out of postures. A yoga strap provides extra length when you're extending your arms or legs. You can place a yoga block under your hands in certain postures until you can reach the floor without it. A blanket provides extra cushion and lift when needed.

Many people experience significant benefits for mind, body, heart, and spirit through yoga. In fact, *yoga* means "union" or "yoke"; it is the integration of all these parts into a unified whole. It can help you learn how to slow down, focus, and listen to your body. It may also help you listen to your heart and soul; you'll stretch literally *and* figuratively!

Keep It Interesting

- In addition to stretching after exercise, periodically set aside time for a head-to-toe stretching session. It will feel so good.

- Listening to music and focusing on your breath can help you relax. When you're relaxed, your body is more responsive to flexibility training.

- Use towels, straps, large balls, and other accessories to add diversity and effectiveness to your stretching.

- Try a stretching class, available on video or DVD or possibly offered by your local fitness facility, community center, or community college. Some classes focus exclusively on flexibility; others combine cardiorespiratory and strength training with stretching.

- Yoga and Pilates are great additions to your regular fitness program. They'll increase your flexibility and strength while teaching you how to focus and calm your mind.

Stretching regularly is a wonderful way to relax while building your flexibility. It will help you tune up while you tune in to your body.

PART 6

Acceptance

Of course, there is no formula for success except, perhaps, an unconditional acceptance of life and what it brings.

—Arthur Rubinstein

CHAPTER 21

Think:
Where Do I Invest
My Energy?

As you free yourself from thinking of foods as good or bad, you can also free yourself from thinking about where you use energy as just exercise and burning calories.

Where you invest your energy is more important than how many calories you burn. When you have diabetes, what should be the natural process of consuming fuel to supply the necessary energy to survive and thrive can consume all of your time and energy. Marlise, from chapter 1, who was caught in a restrictive eating cycle, felt this way:

> When I was diagnosed with diabetes, I dreaded the thought that I would be on a diet for the rest of my life. Now I realize that obsessing about everything I eat leaves me feeling distracted and worried. That's no way to live.

When you're focused on food (or avoiding food), you can't focus on living your life. The primary reason you eat is to fuel your life and provide you with the energy to do whatever you need and want to do. So, what do you want to do? Where do you want to invest your energy?

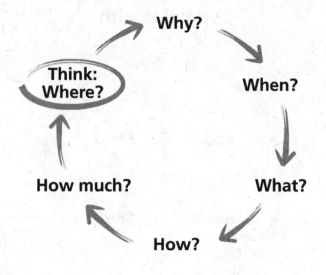

Figure 21.1

The Best Return on Your Investment

You've learned strategies for allowing hunger and fullness to guide your eating again so that you can develop a healthier lifestyle and manage your diabetes without following a rigid diet or exercise regimen. But the most powerful result of freeing yourself from overeating and restrictive eating cycles is that it frees up your energy to focus on what it really takes to make you healthy.

By "healthy," we mean a complete state of physical, intellectual, emotional, and spiritual wellness: health of your body, mind, heart, and spirit. That doesn't mean perfect health; it means *optimal* health: the best health you can have at a certain point in your life given your individual situation. Even though a person with prediabetes or diabetes doesn't have perfect health, it's possible to have optimal health through appropriate medical treatment and self-care, excellent emotional support and coping skills, meaning and purpose in life, and a positive outlook.

Optimal Health

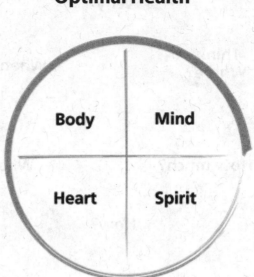

Figure 21.2

Let's take a closer look at these four aspects of your health and where you invest your energy.

Body

When most people think of health, they think of physical health first. Before anything else, your primary needs for shelter, safety, and security must be met. Beyond other basics, like water and enough food for survival, optimal physical health includes nutritious food, an active lifestyle, sufficient rest and sleep, adequate health care, physical touch, and perhaps intimacy. You may also broaden your perspective to include your physical surroundings and the material things in your life. A healthy body and a comfortable physical environment are important because they give you the security and vitality to do what you need and want to do.

Mind

Challenge, growth, creativity, stimulation, and a sense of accomplishment are all important for optimal intellectual health. From a practical standpoint, your thoughts have a powerful impact on your feelings and actions, and therefore your overall health.

Heart

The area of emotional health includes your ability to accurately identify your feelings. This is important because your feelins give you important information about whether what's happening is in alignment with what you really want. Optimal emotional health does not mean being perfectly happy but, rather, embracing the full spectrum of emotions for the depth and richness they bring to your life. Other important aspects of emotional wellness include your ability to cope with your emotions, satisfying relationships with others, effective communication, healthy personal boundaries, and well-developed self-nurturing skills.

Spirit

Spirituality is your sense of connection and purpose. For some this may include religion, but it's really much more than that. It's knowing that who you are is not defined by your possessions, health, appearance, accomplishments, or even contributions. You are worthy of love just as you are. It's the awareness that there is something greater than yourself and that there's a purpose for your life.

Remember Cheryl and Roger from chapter 1? Roger shared these thoughts on what makes him feel healthy:

What I eat affects my physical health, but I can't imagine letting it rule my life. It's more challenging for Cheryl because she has diabetes, but we don't want it to monopolize our attention. I'd rather spend time together and with our friends and try new things. We love to sing in our choir, and we just got a new puppy! What's the point of taking care of your health if you don't take the time to enjoy it?

Invest Your Energy in Optimal Health

Where is your energy going? Where would you like it to go? As you free yourself from overeating and restrictive eating, you can redirect your time and energy toward more productive and satisfying pursuits. As you considered the previous four aspects of your health, perhaps you recognized areas that need more of your attention and energy. Remember, no matter how hard you work in one area, it can't provide the substance of another.

Here are a number of ideas for caring for your physical, intellectual, emotional, and spiritual health. Start with one or two from each category that resonate with you.

Physical Self-Care

- Focus on improving your health rather than a number on the scale.

- Make small changes rather than trying to overhaul your entire life. If needed, work your way through this book again, one chapter at a time.

- Be careful not to turn this into a diet by trying to follow it perfectly or feeling guilty when you don't; perfection is not necessary for becoming healthier.

- Check your blood glucose regularly and share your blood glucose log with your health care team. Keep your diabetes care card up to date (review chapter 14).

- Choose a personal physician and have regular checkups. Take care of your preventive health needs and don't ignore new, persistent, or unusual symptoms.

- Eat fresh, healthful, and interesting foods.

- Engage in regular, enjoyable physical activity.

- Limit your screen time. Instead of spending passive hours in front of the television or computer, do something active that restores your energy.

- Get plenty of rest and adequate sleep so you'll feel clear and refreshed.

- Give and receive physical affection.

- Treat yourself to a massage, manicure, pedicure, or facial.

- Take a hot bath or long shower to relax and unwind.

- Wear comfortable clothes that fit your current size and shape.

- Clear the physical clutter around you.

- Create a pleasant personal space for yourself. Include comfortable pillows, photographs, candles, music, or whatever makes you feel happy and calm.

- Plant a garden and grow fresh vegetables, herbs, or flowers.

- Spend time in nature walking, hiking, camping, or just sitting.

Intellectual Self-Care

- Lay a firm foundation by examining your values and priorities.

- Give your brain a map to follow by setting inspiring short- and long-term goals. Visualize yourself reaching your goals daily.

- Recognize that your thoughts lead to your feelings, actions, and results. Challenge yourself to think positively and powerfully.

- Learn something new: a skill, trade, hobby, language, or anything else you find interesting.

- Read often and experience new genres outside of your usual preferences. For example, if you usually read romance novels, try mysteries or classic literature.

- Travel or explore areas close to home, such as museums or other novel places.

- Do brainteasers and play challenging games, alone and with others.

- Be creative, especially if you don't ordinarily have an opportunity to express yourself creatively. Experiment with art, crafts, and hobbies.

- Listen to music, sing, or play an instrument.

- Take classes online or at your local community center or college.

- Become an expert in something. Learn everything you can about an area and share that knowledge with others by writing, speaking, or teaching.

- Explore new occupational and career opportunities.

Emotional Self-Care

- Love yourself as you are right now.

- Identify your emotions through writing in a journal or talking with a trusted friend or counselor.

- Spend quality time with your family and friends, having fun and sharing. Build intimacy and emotional connections with your partner. Make new friends and renew old friendships.

- Set appropriate boundaries with others. By letting other people know how far into your emotional space they can go, you'll build healthier relationships.

- Assert yourself to let others know how you feel, what you think, and what you need. Accept that beyond that, you can't control what other people think, feel, or do.

- Manage stress effectively. It's not possible or even desirable to eliminate stress, but you can learn to release and cope with it.

- Practice forgiveness. Harboring anger and hurt is harmful and eats up precious emotional energy.

- Be vulnerable. Let people you trust see your imperfections and fears. This can deepen intimacy and free you from the need to be perfect.

- Seek coaching, counseling, or therapy if needed for emotional support and to build coping skills.

Spiritual Self-Care

- Practice mindfulness. Be fully present in whatever you're doing—eating, talking, working, or playing—to experience the full pleasure and meaning.

- Renew and restore yourself through prayer and meditation.

- Schedule time for your inner work. Know yourself, your values, your dreams, and your purpose. Define your guiding principles so that you'll have a clear path to follow.

- See your problems as opportunities for learning and growth.

- Reclaim your joy! Experiencing joy is possible even as you face challenges.

- Look for the good in others; it's there somewhere just waiting to be discovered.

- Volunteer and give back to your community by helping others.

- Visit your place of worship (or find one).

- Read meaningful, inspirational works.

- Have an attitude of gratitude. Being thankful for even the smallest of things will remind you of all that you have.

- Practice kindness without any expectation of receiving something in return. Remember, you already have everything you need to live an abundant life.

Strategies: Balance, Variety, and Moderation in All Things

As you consider where you invest your energy, you may realize you've been neglecting an aspect of your physical, intellectual, emotional, or spiritual life. If you made a long mental to-do list, let it go. Ann had a new twist on it:

As I raced around, trying to get my house cleaned before we left on vacation, it dawned on me that the principles of "balance, variety, and moderation" don't just apply to food. They apply to life. Whether I'm working, exercising, cleaning, playing, or socializing, I get myself in over my head, and I start to feel exhausted and frustrated. Instead, I'm going to seek balance in how I spend my time, variety in my exercise and playtime, and moderation in my work, both at the office and at home.

Mindful Energy Management

Self-care is not about spending an equal amount of time or energy in each area. It's about making the commitment to care for yourself and meet your true needs. Make conscious personal choices about how you'll deal with the multitude of responsibilities, stressors, and opportunities you face. It worked for Sara:

Until now, I was eating on a schedule, never allowing myself to get hungry. Last night I found myself rummaging through the cabinet, looking for something to fill me up. When I realized what I was doing, I paused and asked myself, Am I hungry? I wasn't, so I knew I needed something besides food.

I remembered all the digital photos that I had been meaning to organize. I turned on some music, sat down in front of my computer, and spent hours filing all the photos by year and event. I even made CDs of the best pictures to give to each of my children and grandchildren on their birthdays. The thought of food didn't cross my mind the whole evening. I didn't need to eat; I needed to create! And for the first time in a long time, I truly felt full.

Decide where you'll invest your energy—body, mind, heart, and spirit—to create a truly healthy lifestyle. You'll finally break free from your eat-repent-repeat cycle when food serves its true purpose: fueling your full and satisfying life.

CHAPTER 22

Care:
A Flexible Approach
to Self-Care

There's a saying: "Expecting yourself and others to be perfect guarantees that you'll never be satisfied." Letting go of the need to get it right and, instead, approaching your eating with flexibility and self-acceptance is the beginning of a transformation that will ripple through all aspects of your life.

What to Do When You Get Offtrack (Hint: It's Normal!)

At this point, you may be asking yourself, *What now?* You may even be a little concerned that you'll return to old habits if that is what happened in the past. Unlike following rigid rules, which gets harder and harder over time, learning to manage your diabetes mindfully becomes easier with practice. Simply choose to use every opportunity to learn more about yourself and why, when, what, how, and how much you eat—as well as where you invest your energy.

Don't expect yourself to be perfect. It isn't possible or even necessary. You're in charge. Whenever you recognize that you are offtrack, notice the decision point where you are in your eating cycle and return to instinctive eating with your next decision. Look at the following examples and review the mindful eating cycle (figure 1.1) to see how this works.

Back to Instinctive Eating

Learning opportunity 1. *In the middle of eating, I notice I'm eating too fast.*

> **Why?** *I've been conscious about eating instinctively to meet my needs for fuel, nourishment, and enjoyment. I was in my instinctive eating cycle when I started eating.*
>
> **When?** *I was at level 2 on the Hunger and Fullness Scale when I decided to eat.*
>
> **What?** *I chose tasty, healthy food that I really wanted.*
>
> **How?** *I paused when I hit my speed bump, and I noticed how fast I was eating. I'm reading my mail while eating. I'm distracted, so I'm not eating with intention or attention.*
>
> **Back to instinctive eating:** *I'll stop reading my mail until I'm finished eating. I'll slow down and focus on enjoying my food.*

Learning opportunity 2. *I've been overeating snacks and sweets all week at work.*

> **Why?** *I'd been more mindful about my eating for several months, so my blood glucose had been on target. I saw something on TV about avoiding all "white foods," like sugar and flour. I knew it was a mistake but thought it might be worth a try. Before I knew it, I had slipped back into my restrictive eating cycle.*
>
> **When?** *I was trying to eat when hungry but was craving foods I thought I had stopped having problems with.*
>
> **What?** *I was trying to avoid flour and sugar—but that seems to be all I think about now.*
>
> **Back to instinctive eating:** *Clearly, trying to follow a rigid plan increased my desire for those foods. Instead of restricting myself, I went back to eating what I love in moderation and paying attention to hunger and fullness. My cravings decreased almost immediately.*

Learning Opportunity 3. *I notice that my blood glucose has been out of target.*

> **Why?** *I've slipped back into an overeating cycle.*

When? *I haven't been asking myself Am I hungry? because I know that most of the time the answer is no but I want to eat anyway. I guess something is out of balance and driving my overeating, but until now I never took the time to think or do anything about it.*

Back to instinctive eating: *I remembered how good it felt when I really listened to my body and practiced self-care. I started doing my body-mind-heart scan whenever I wanted to eat. It quickly became clear that I feel stretched too thin and have been rewarding myself with food. Instead of beating myself up for overeating, I made a list of things I can do to nurture myself: read an article from a favorite magazine, meditate, take a hot bath, ask for help, start planning my next vacation. I already feel better and less like overeating.*

Strategies: Measuring Change

Take a look at how far you've come. On a sheet of paper, draw a vertical line. At the top write, "Flexible," and at the bottom, write, "Rigid." Then draw a horizontal line intersecting the vertical line through the middle. On the right side, write, "Self-Care," and on the left, write, "Neglect."

Using the following explanations, think about where you were when you started this process, and place yourself in one of the four quadrants. Then think about where you are now and, again, place yourself in a quadrant.

Measuring Change

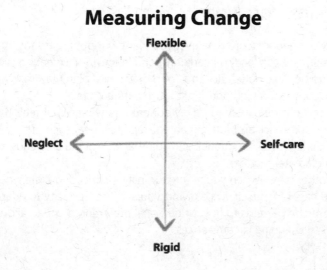

Figure 22.1

Self-Care vs. Neglect

On the horizontal line, think about how the decisions you make affect your health and well-being. At one end of the spectrum is self-care. Decisions that promote self-care have the most desirable effects on your physical, intellectual, emotional, and spiritual health. Obvious examples include eating a healthy diet, exercising regularly, and checking your blood glucose, but also consider other ways you care for your body, mind, heart, and spirit.

On the other end of the spectrum is neglect. You're neglecting yourself when your decisions ignore or disregard your best interests. Examples of neglect include eating an excessive amount of saturated fat–containing foods or eating too much even though it raises your blood glucose.

Flexible vs. Rigid

On the vertical line, think about how you make your day-to-day decisions. At one end of the spectrum is flexibility. Flexibility allows you to adapt to any situation. Another way of thinking about flexibility is freedom, meaning that you can make any decision you choose at any given time.

At the other end of the spectrum is rigidity. Rigid decision making is strict, with no room for error or unexpected detours. When you try to rigidly follow a diet, for example, you strive to be perfect, not allowing yourself to make any mistakes or to ever go "off the plan."

Where Are You Now?

The flexibility or freedom to do whatever you want without regard for your best interests or self-care can lead to overeating and inactivity (overeating cycle). At the other extreme, rigid adherence to a food or exercise plan may improve your health, but it comes at a high price (restrictive eating cycle).

Since it's nearly impossible to rigidly adhere to any plan that feels harsh or restrictive, you shift back and forth in an eat-repent-repeat cycle. This neglects your physical, intellectual, emotional, and spiritual well-being and leads to guilt, shame, and, ultimately, defeat.

On the other hand, when you're in your instinctive eating cycle, you strive to take good care of yourself while giving yourself the flexibility to adapt your eating and exercise patterns to fit your personal preferences and to allow yourself to adjust to changing circumstances.

Where Are You Now?

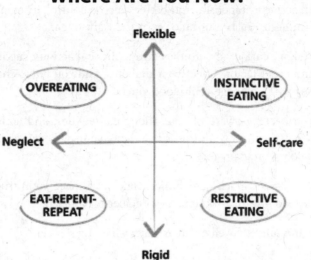

Figure 22.2

Where do you want to be in the future? What do you need to work on to achieve that vision of yourself?

A Lifelong Approach

By practicing flexible self-care, you create a pattern of eating and living that you can maintain for life:

- You listen to your internal cues of hunger and satisfaction instead of trying to follow strict or arbitrary rules about your eating.

- You build a strong foundation of nutritional information and choose from all foods freely to meet your needs instead of trying every fad diet that comes along.

- You eat foods you really enjoy without guilt instead of depriving yourself or bingeing.

- You eat mindfully, in a manner that nourishes your body, mind, and spirit, instead of eating unconsciously or obsessing over every bite.

- You're physically active because it gives you energy, stress relief, an active metabolism, and better glucose control, instead of exercising to punish yourself or earn the right to eat.

- You are curious about how eating, physical activity, medications, and other factors affect your diabetes, and you make changes as needed to manage your blood glucose.

- You become aware of your thoughts, feelings, and actions and how they affect you instead of judging yourself because you didn't follow a program perfectly.

- You create a self-care buffer zone and meet your true needs instead of eating too much or neglecting yourself.

Mark and Julie are well on their way to lifelong self-care:

We both love to eat and thought that having diabetes would be the end of our enjoyment. But now we're healthier and enjoying food even more. Julie took a cooking class for diabetes at the community college and makes amazing meals with loads of fresh vegetables. Not to be outdone, I built a barbecue, and Julie loves my grilled salmon with papaya salsa. I'm not saying we don't still love chocolate cake, but now we go out to dinner and share an entrée and one piece of cake, and it's plenty. I think the biggest difference is in our awareness of why we're eating and how our food choices affect not only our blood glucose levels but also how we feel.

CHAPTER 23

Nourish:
Putting It All Together

W e've covered a lot of ground in learning how to manage your diabetes mindfully. This chapter will pull all of this information together to help you plan your meals and snacks for optimal health and enjoyment.

Mindful Eating with Diabetes

Even without diabetes, there's a lot to think about when planning your meals. To simplify the process, let's return to the mindful eating cycle and review some of the key points covered in other chapters to help you focus on the important decisions to consider when planning your meals.

Why do I eat? When you know why, everything else falls into place. When your primary reason for eating is to fuel your body for optimal health, your meal is both nourishing and enjoyable. When you have diabetes, you also eat to manage your blood glucose and minimize your risk of complications.

When do I eat? Becoming mindful of your body's hunger signals lets you know when to eat. The Hunger and Fullness Scale helps you identify different levels of hunger. If you're at risk for hypoglycemia, noticing that you're hungry can help you identify decreasing blood glucose before it drops to a dangerously low level. When you have diabetes, your blood glucose level also helps you assess your fuel needs. The key is to be sure to have food available to eat when you're hungry (and glucose tabs or gel if you're at risk for hypoglycemia).

What do I eat? Remind yourself that all foods can fit into a healthy diet—even when you have diabetes. Visualize your plate as we described in chapter 7 and ask these three questions to help you choose delicious and nutritious snacks and meals:

> *What do I want?* Recognizing what you're hungry for helps you make satisfying choices.
>
> *What do I need?* Use these three principles—balance, variety, and moderation—to decide what to eat:
>
> > *Balance:* Balance your intake with your output for glucose and weight management, and balance eating for nourishment with eating for enjoyment for a sustainable healthy lifestyle.
> >
> > *Variety:* Eat a variety of foods to meet your nutritional requirements and prevent monotony for overall health and enjoyment.
> >
> > *Moderation:* When your goal is to feel good after eating, you're more likely to eat wisely and moderately.
>
> *What do I have?* With diabetes, it's important to take responsibility for keeping food on hand to eat when you're hungry so that you're not dependent on the environment. When you know what you want and need, you can choose a snack or meal that is satisfying and provides needed nutrients and just the right amount of carbohydrate to prevent your blood glucose from dropping too low or swinging too high.

How do I eat? Mindful eating—eating with intention and attention—increases your enjoyment and satisfaction with your meal. Remember that mindful eating begins with awareness of your physical state, thoughts, and feelings. It also includes the selection and preparation of your food. During eating, you'll want to stay aware of the appearance, aroma, flavors, and textures of your food, as well as your satiety signals to help you determine when you've had enough.

How much do I eat? Mindfulness helps you recognize your satiety and fullness signals, but it's important to also consider how much you're eating in terms of your nutrient intake. When considering how much to eat, think about your intake at each meal or snack as well as your total daily intake.

Where do I invest my energy? Physical activity and exercise are important for glucose and weight management. The "Live" chapters describe the benefits of increasing your stamina, strength, and flexibility. The last "Think" chapter also explores the importance of investing your energy in caring for your body, mind, heart, and spirit.

Balancing Your Plate

Review the plate-planning strategies you learned in chapter 7, and apply the nutrition information you read in the "Nourish" chapters. Choose foods that support your overall health goals. The following tables may help you make healthier choices.

Using the plate-planning method, you could select 1 cup of broccoli, 1 cup of cauliflower, 1 cup of white rice with 2 teaspoons of butter, 3 ounces of pan-fried steak, and a glass of milk for dinner. This meal has three carbohydrate choices (approximately 60 grams of carbohydrate); 8 grams of fiber from the vegetables; and protein from the meat and milk. You could boost your fiber intake by 4 grams by choosing brown rice. Fat in this meal comes from the butter, steak, and milk; by using a lean cooking method such as grilling, and choosing margarine (without trans fat) and skim milk, you could decrease the amount of saturated fat in the meal. You could add omega 3 fatty acids by choosing 4 ounces of salmon as your protein.

Breakfast using this method might include 1 slice of whole grain toast with 2 teaspoons of margarine (without trans fat), half of a grapefruit, and a container of light yogurt. This meal has about 45 grams of carbohydrate and 5 grams of fiber. Another example of breakfast is 1 cup of cooked oatmeal made with 8 ounces of 1 percent milk and topped with 3/4 cup of blueberries and 2 tablespoons of sliced almonds. This is four carbohydrate choices (60 grams of carbohydrate); 13 grams of fiber from the oatmeal, blueberries, and nuts; protein and a small amount of saturated fat in the milk; and a small amount of protein and polyunsaturated fat in the almonds.

Making Healthier Choices

Foods That Contain Little Carbohydrate

Low-Carbohydrate Vegetables

Fresh or Frozen:
Beets, broccoli, carrots, cauliflower, celery, cucumbers, eggplant, green beans,
green-leafy vegetables (beet greens, collard greens, kale, lettuce, spinach,
Swiss chard), mushrooms, okra, onions, peppers, squash (spaghetti, summer,
zucchini), turnips

Protein

Grill, Broil, Boil or Bake:
Skinless chicken or turkey, trimmed of visible fat
Fish and shellfish: baked, boiled, broiled
Lean beef (loin, shoulder, leg) trimmed of visible fat
Lean, ground beef, drained
Lean pork (loin, shoulder, leg)
Eggs, egg whites (2), low-fat egg substitute
Soy (tofu, edamame, meat substitutes)

Fat

Replace solid fat with oil (vegetable, canola, olive, or peanut oil)
Avocado, hummus, nuts, and nut butters (peanut butter)
Lite or reduced fat mayonnaise, dressings, cream cheese, or sour cream
Healthier cooking methods: Nonstick pans or cooking spray,
cooking in water or broth
Serve dressing and sauces on the side
Eat fish high in omega-3 fatty acids (mackerel, salmon, and tuna)
Avoid trans fat

Foods That Contain Carbohydrate

Grains, Starchy Vegetables and Beans

Whole-grain bread, bagels, English muffins
Brown or wild rice, couscous, quinoa
Whole-wheat pasta, blended wheat pasta
Cold whole-grain cereals, such as shredded wheat
Hot whole-grain cereal, such as oatmeal
100% whole-wheat or corn tortillas
Whole-grain: crackers, flatbread, melba toast, popcorn
Parsnips, potato - baked or boiled (white or sweet)
Winter squash
Fresh or frozen corn
Fresh or frozen peas
Beans

Fruit

High-fiber fruit: fresh fruit with skin and peels
(apples, grapes, peaches, pears, plums),
berries (blackberries, blueberries, raspberries, strawberries),
citrus (clementines, grapefruit, oranges), kiwi, mangoes, papaya
Frozen or canned fruit (with no added sugar or syrup)

Dairy

Skim (nonfat) milk, 1% milk
Low-fat or nonfat yogurt with less than 20 grams of carbohydrate

Figure 23.1

Experimenting with Food and Blood Glucose

The purpose of meal planning is to help keep your blood glucose in the target range after meals (fasting or before meals: 70 to 130 mg/dL; two hours after eating: <180 mg/dL). To determine if your dietary changes are successful, conduct some experiments to help you figure out how different types and amounts of food affect your blood glucose. For these experiments, you'll need the following: food, your blood glucose monitor, your blood glucose log, and your awareness. For each experiment, write down your hunger and fullness level and check your blood glucose before the meal or snack. To keep it simple, make one change at a time (see below). Write down your choices so you'll remember what you ate. Note your hunger and fullness level within thirty minutes after eating. Recheck your blood glucose two hours after eating.

Experiment 1: What happens when you eat different amounts of carbohydrate? For this experiment, fill half your plate with low-carbohydrate vegetables and a quarter of your plate with a serving of protein. For the upper-right section of your meal, select your usual amount of carbohydrate-containing food. If you are physically comfortable after eating (not still hungry and not too full) and your blood glucose is in your target range—less than 180 mg/dL two hours after eating—then you'll know that your body responded well to that amount of carbohydrate.

If your blood glucose is above target—over 180 mg/dL two hours after eating—conduct additional experiments to see what happens when you decrease the amount of carbohydrate you eat by reducing your portion sizes or the number of carbohydrate-containing foods you eat. Try three to four servings of carbohydrate-containing foods, such as starchy vegetables, grains or grain products, fruit, dairy, or some combination of these food groups. (If you plan to have dessert, save one or two of your carbohydrate choices.) If you feel comfortable counting carbohydrates, aim for a total of 45 or 60 grams.

Experiment 2: What happens to your blood glucose when you eat different types of food in the same meal? Once you have a pretty good idea of how different amounts of carbohydrate affect your blood glucose, you can experiment with manipulating other foods in your meal. For example, eating a mixture of carbohydrate, fiber, and protein may help stabilize your blood glucose (hold it steady), preventing unexpected drops. Think of this as changing a mountain with jagged peaks into rolling hills.

For example, a breakfast of white toast, skim milk, and juice is primarily carbohydrate. If you still feel hungry or your blood glucose is elevated two hours after eating, adding fiber, protein, or fat (preferably oils rather than solid fat) to your meal may help. You could add fiber by making your toast with high-fiber bread, substituting a high-fiber cereal, or swapping the juice for whole fruit, such as blueberries or strawberries. You could add protein and fat by putting peanut butter on your toast or adding an egg.

Experiment 3: What happens when you add protein to a snack of carbohydrate? If you typically eat carbohydrates like crackers, fruit, or sweets for a snack, check your hunger and fullness level thirty minutes after eating and your blood glucose two hours after your meal and record your results. Repeat once or twice. Then experiment by adding protein to your snack. For example, you might have hummus with crackers, cottage cheese and sliced peaches, or a small handful of almonds and an ounce of chocolate chips. You can try this same experiment by adding healthy fat to your snack. For example, you could add one tablespoon of sunflower seeds to yogurt or mash a quarter of an avocado with salsa to make guacamole to serve with corn tortilla chips.

With experimentation, you'll find the best mixture of foods for your blood glucose and satiety levels. Here's what Jane said:

> After meeting with my dietitian, I started pairing my carbohydrates with foods that are supposed to slow the rise of blood glucose. I was so happy with the results. I added sliced chicken to stir-fried vegetables, black olives to my salad, and walnuts to my yogurt. I felt more satisfied, and most of the time I didn't need a snack between meals anymore.

CHAPTER 24

Live:
Mindful Movement

J ust as it is essential to balance eating for nourishment with eating for enjoyment, it's important that you find physical activities that are both challenging and enjoyable. Mindful movement guides you to do what you love and love what you do as part of your overall self-care and diabetes management.

Do What You Love

Before joining another gym, dragging out your stationary bike, or buying new walking shoes, maximize your likelihood of choosing the right activities for your personality. Your awareness of your preferences will help you decide what types of physical activity you're most likely to enjoy and stick with.

Why?

1. My main motivation for exercising is to:

    a. look better

    b. feel better

    c. be healthier

    d. other: _____

2. I am motivated by rewards like:

   a. visual graphs and numbers

   b. money or prizes

   c. intangibles, such as increased energy or better sleep

   d. other: _____

It's important to identify your reasons for exercising and set your fitness goals using positive, powerful, measurable terms to keep yourself focused and inspired. Be specific about the results you want and the rewards you'll receive when you achieve your goals. For example, if you're motivated to become healthier and you like to see tangible results, you could make a graph that tracks your resting heart rate, blood pressure, and fasting blood glucose. If looking better is your goal and you like prizes, you could pay yourself a dollar every time you work out to save up to buy yourself new clothing. Even if you enjoy less-tangible rewards, be specific about the results you're looking for, like *I have enough energy to play with my grandchildren.*

When?

1. I feel most energetic and alert in the:

   a. morning

   b. afternoon

   c. evening

2. In the past, exercise has worked best:

   a. when I do it early in the day before other things get in my way

   b. when I do it at work during my breaks or lunch hour

   c. when I stop at the gym on my way home so I don't have to go back out again

   d. when I do it after dinner to unwind or when I have help with the kids

Plan your workouts during your peak energy times, when you're most likely to do it. Make it easier on yourself by scheduling a time that's most convenient.

What?

1. I am:
   a. easily bored
   b. a creature of habit

2. I really like:
   a. technical gadgets, like monitors and tracking programs
   b. a real physical workout so I don't have to think about anything
   c. creative or artistic expression

3. When it comes to competition:
   a. I feel stressed
   b. I like to challenge myself
   c. a little is healthy and fun
   d. I am very competitive

There are many different forms of physical activity, so the challenge is to find several types that suit your preferences. If you're a gadget guru, you might like a fancy pedometer or gyms equipped with high-tech monitors to track your progress on all the machines. If you like artistic expression, you may enjoy dance or yoga. If you thrive on competition, look for team sports or competitive events, like races; you can also challenge competitive friends to play racquetball, tennis, or other sports. If you enjoy challenging yourself, set goals and consider purchasing devices that help you monitor incremental changes. If you don't like competition but like to be with others, look for classes and gyms with a supportive environment.

Respect your personal exercise traits and experiment with different activities until you find a perfect fit.

How?

1. Time for exercise:
    a. is not a problem
    b. is a challenge but can be arranged when I make it a priority
    c. is last on my list

2. I'd exercise more if it wasn't for:
    a. the time it takes to get to the gym and back
    b. family commitments
    c. work
    d. the cost of gym membership or equipment

3. I stay on track best when:
    a. I set a goal to work out most days of the week but stay flexible about when
    b. I write my workout schedule in my appointment calendar
    c. I know someone else is expecting me to be there

4. When I decide to do something:
    a. I have a hard time getting started
    b. I stick with it unless it becomes inconvenient
    c. I make it happen no matter what

The reality is that making the commitment to invest time, money, and energy in becoming more active isn't easy. When you know what makes it easier and anticipate what could get in your way, you can plan to work around those challenges. For example, if you're concerned about taking time away from your family, you could involve them in your workouts, exercise during your workday, or decide that the time it takes will pay off because you'll be healthier and less stressed.

Who?

1. I prefer to be:
   a. by myself
   b. with a friend or partner
   c. in a group where I know everyone
   d. anonymous in a crowd

2. I need:
   a. to exercise at my own pace
   b. the support of a friend or partner
   c. the accountability of showing up to a class or lesson
   d. to be pushed by a trainer or teacher

If you prefer to be alone, choose activities like walking, biking, or using exercise videos. If you enjoy being with one or two others, invite someone to walk, hike, play tennis, or go to the gym with you. If you enjoy socializing while exercising, consider joining a sports team, signing up for a class, or arranging classes at church or work. If you prefer to work out with strangers, join a large gym for weight training, spin classes, or other group exercise. If you need accountability and support, sign up for a class, or find a workout buddy or personal trainer to come to your home or meet you at the gym. Mix it up depending on your mood.

Where?

1. I love to be:
   a. at home
   b. outdoors
   c. in an exercise environment

2. When people look at me:

   a. I'm self-conscious and embarrassed

   b. I just ignore them

   c. I'm flattered

If you enjoy being at home, use exercise videos or websites, a treadmill, a stationary bike, or a home gym. If you're more of an outdoors type, you'll enjoy walking, hiking, bike riding, or sports. If you need a designated exercise space and don't mind having other people around, join a gym or studio.

Love What You Do

Moving mindfully—in other words, choosing and doing physical activity with *intention* and *attention*—guides you to do activities you love and love the activities you do.

Move with intention. Be purposeful when you choose your activities.

- Choose activities that suit your personality and mood.

- Choose activities that meet your body's needs.

- Move with the goal of feeling better afterward.

Move with attention. Be attentive during your activities.

- Become aware of your surroundings, physical sensations, thoughts, and feelings.

- Listen to your body's cues of intensity, discomfort, and fatigue.

- Appreciate your body's stamina, flexibility, and strength.

When you move with the intention of caring for yourself, you'll choose activities that you find challenging and enjoyable. When you're attentive, you'll appreciate your body's capacity to become stronger and healthier. Let's look at each of these attributes in more detail.

Moving with Intention

As you learned to be in charge of what you eat, you asked yourself three questions: *What do I want? What do I need?* and *What do I have?* These questions can also help you choose the best physical activity at any given time.

What do I want to do? *What do I feel like doing (if anything)? Am I in the mood to be more active or in the mood for structured exercise? Do I want to do housework, work in my garden, walk my dog, or play with my kids? What does my body feel like doing right now—cardio, strength training, or stretching?*

What do I need to do? *What have I been doing this week? Am I due for a rest, or do I need to get moving somehow today? Have I met the goals I set for my personal fitness prescription? What's missing from my program recently? Does my physical activity reflect balance, variety, and moderation?*

What do I have to do? *What are my options for activity? What equipment, classes, or other activities are available to me? What does my time and schedule allow? What's the weather like? Do I want to go to the gym, be outside, or do something at home? Is there someone I could exercise with?*

Strategies: Body-Mind-Heart Scan during Exercise

Just as the body-mind-heart scan helps you identify hunger, fullness, and other sensations, thoughts, and feelings, it will help you become more aware of the full experience of being physically active.

1. *Presence:* Get centered. Tune in to the experience and become aware of your body and surroundings. Pay attention to the sights, sounds, aromas, weather, and other people in your environment.

2. *Body:* Connect with your physical sensations. Tune in to your breath, heart rate, and other sensations. How does your body feel as you move? How do different activities and intensities feel? What do you need to do to make it more comfortable, challenging, or enjoyable?

223

3. *Mind:* What thoughts are running through your mind? What feelings are your thoughts creating? How are your thoughts affecting your experience with this activity?

4. *Heart:* Become aware of your emotions. What feelings do you have about exercising? Are you having fun or feeling punished? Are you enjoying the atmosphere, the other people, and the experience?

Moving with Attention

There may be times when you feel like watching television while doing floor exercises or reading a magazine while riding a stationary bike. Distracting yourself or multitasking may have its place, but it can also diminish your ability to have a complete mind-body experience. Choosing to move more mindfully increases your awareness of your body, which decreases your risk of injury and boredom and increases your enjoyment and ability to optimize the time you invest. Further, mindfulness during activity has a calming, meditative effect that carries over into other aspects of your life.

Mindful Movement

Experiment with the following methods to be more mindful during activity:

Intentional practice. Before starting, set an intention for your session that gives you a focus to return to throughout. For example, your intention might be to stay connected to your breath, challenge yourself in some of the poses or exercises, or express gratitude throughout your session.

Meditative walking. Inhale slowly for four steps, hold your breath for one step, exhale slowly for four steps, and then hold for one step. Repeat. Experiment with different lengths to see what works best for you.

Environmental awareness. As you walk, cycle, or jog, stay aware of the details in your environment: the sights, the sounds, the weather, and so forth. You can even make it part of your training; for example, choose a beautiful tree in the distance and pick up your pace until you reach it.

Gratitude attitude. A powerful technique is to think of everything you're grateful for as you walk. Imagine a ripple that moves outward. Start by expressing gratitude for everything about yourself: your body, mind, heart, and spirit. Then express gratitude for those around you: your family, friends, coworkers, and so on. Then move on to other things you are grateful for: where you live, the weather, the cultural events in your city—you get the idea.

Move mindfully. Yoga, tai chi, qigong, and Pilates are taught with an emphasis on mindfulness. As you notice your awareness and thoughts drift elsewhere, gently return your focus to the present moment.

Centering breath. Matching your movement to your breath is a powerful centering tool because it requires focus and awareness. Tie slow, deep breaths to your movements so that each movement begins and ends precisely with the start and finish of the breath. For example, open your arms slowly overhead as you inhale, and then lower them back to your sides as you exhale.

Breath awareness. To ensure both mindfulness and proper movement during strength training, exhale slowly as you shorten or contract the muscle (for example, lifting your leg), and inhale slowly as you lengthen or relax the muscle (for example, lowering your leg).

Technique focus. When you learn a new activity, such as ballroom dancing, tennis, or swimming, you necessarily become more mindful of your body, movements, and technique.

Muscle focus. Bring your awareness and attention to the muscle group you are working, ensuring that you're doing the exercise primarily with that muscle group. For example, while doing an abdominal crunch, focus on the contraction in the front and center of your abdomen. Be sure you aren't using your hands behind your head to pull you up or relying on momentum to swing your body up and down.

Counting. Count as you do repetitions to ensure slow, steady movement: 1, 2, 3 as you shorten; 1, 2, 3 as you lengthen.

Nonjudgmental awareness. Become curious about your thoughts and feelings as you move into different poses or exercises. Without judgment, notice whether thoughts like *my favorite pose* or *I hate this one* make the activity more or less enjoyable. Practice disconnecting from those habitual thoughts and opinions by focusing on your breath.

Becoming more intentional about your thoughts, feelings, and choices of activities will help you discover what inspires, challenges, and rewards you. Becoming more attentive helps you appreciate the privilege of moving your body, allowing you to experience the joy of being fully present in the moment. In this way, exercise is no longer a means to an end but an end in itself.

Whether you are moving, eating, or managing your diabetes mindfully, we wish you peace and joy in your journey!

Resources

Diabetes

- Diabetes and Mindful Eating, our website and blog: www.diabetesandmindfuleating.com

- Fearless Blood Glucose Monitoring Log, available at our "Resources" web page: www.diabetesandmindfuleating.com/resources.html

- Diabetes Care Card, available at our "Resources" web page: www.diabetesandmindfuleating.com/resources.html

- American Diabetes Association: www.diabetes.org

Fitness

- National Institute on Aging *Exercise & Physical Activity* guide: www.nia.nih.gov/HealthInformation/Publications/ExerciseGuide or available by phone at 1-800-222-2225

- Illustrations of strength and flexibility exercises: *Eat What You Love, Love What You Eat: How to Break Your Eat-Repent-Repeat Cycle* by Michelle May, M.D. (Am I Hungry? Publishing, 2011)

- Exercise Is Medicine: www.exerciseismedicine.org/keys.htm

Mindful Eating

- Am I Hungry? ® Mindful Eating Workshops And Facilitator Training Program: www.amihungry.com

- The Center for Mindful Eating: www.tcme.org

- Resources for Professionals Using Mindful Eating: www.megrette.com

Nutrition

- U.S. Department of Health and Human Services Dietary Guidelines: www.health.gov/Dietaryguidelines/

- U.S. Department of Agriculture: www.choosemyplate.gov

- How to Read a Nutrition Label, available at our "Resources" web page: www.diabetesandmindfuleating.com/resources.html

- Academy of Nutrition and Dietetics (formerly the American Dietetic Association): www.eatright.org

- American Dietetic Association, food exchange lists/carb content of common foods: www.eatright.org/HealthProfessionals/content .aspx?id=101

References

American Association of Clinical Endocrinologists (AACE) Medical Guidelines for Clinical Practice for the Management of Diabetes Mellitus. 2007a. "5. Hypertension Management: Section 5.2.3. Pharmacology and Mechanisms of Action of Antihypertensive Agents." *Endocrine Practice* 13 (Suppl. 1):35–38.

———. 2007b. "6. Lipid Management: 6.1. Executive Summary." *Endocrine Practice* 13 (Suppl. 1):40.

American College of Sports Medicine (ACSM). 2006. *ACSM's Resource Manual for Guidelines for Exercise Testing and Prescription.* 5th ed. Baltimore: Lippincott Williams & Wilkins.

American College of Sports Medicine (ACSM) and the American Diabetes Association (ADA). 2010. "Exercise and Type 2 Diabetes: American College of Sports Medicine and the American Diabetes Association—Joint Position Statement." *Medicine and Science in Sports and Exercise* 42 (12):2282–303.

American Diabetes Association (ADA). 2008. "Nutrition Recommendations and Interventions for Diabetes." *Diabetes Care* 31 (Suppl. 1):S61-78.

American Diabetes Association (ADA). 2011. "Standards of Medical Care in Diabetes—2011." *Diabetes Care* 34 (Suppl. 1):S11–61. doi:10.2337/dc11-S011.

Bojanowska, E., and A. Nowak. 2007. "Interactions between Leptin and Exendin-4, a Glucagon-Like Peptide-1 Agonist, in the Regulation of Food Intake in the Rat." *Journal of Physiology and Pharmacology* 58 (2):349–60.

Brewer, K. W., H. P. Chase, S. Owen, and S. K. Garg. 1998. "Slicing the Pie: Correlating HbA1c Values with Average Blood Glucose Values in a Pie Chart Form." *Diabetes Care* 21 (2):209–12.

Centers for Disease Control and Prevention (CDC). 2011. "National Diabetes Fact Sheet: National Estimates and General Information on Diabetes and Prediabetes in the United States, 2011." Atlanta, GA: U.S. Department of Health and Human Services, Centers for Disease Control and Prevention.

Ciampolini, M., and R. Biachi. 2006. "Training to Estimate Blood Glucose and to Form Associations with Initial Hunger." *Nutrition and Metabolism* 3:42.

Ciampolini, M., D. Lovell-Smith, R. Bianchi, B. de Pont, M. Sifone, M. van Weeren, W. de Hahn, L. Borselli, and A. Pietrobelli. 2010. "Sustained Self-Regulation of Energy Intake: Initial Hunger Improves Insulin Sensitivity." *Journal of Nutrition and Metabolism.* doi:10.1155/2010/286952.

Ciampolini, M., D. Lovell-Smith, and M. Sifone. 2010. "Sustained Self-Regulation of Energy Intake: Loss of Weight in Overweight Subjects, Maintenance of Weight in Normal-Weight Subjects." *Nutrition and Metabolism* 7:4.

Cummings, S., E. S. Parham, and G. Strain. 2002. "Position of the American Dietetic Association: Weight Management." *Journal of the American Dietetic Association* 102 (8):1145–55.

Gannon, M. C., and F. Q. Nuttall. 2006. "Control of Blood Glucose in Type 2 Diabetes without Weight Loss by Modification of Diet Composition." *Nutrition and Metabolism* 3:16. doi:10.1186/1743-7075-3-16.

Gerstein, D. E., G. Woodward-Lopez, A. E. Evans, K. Kelsey, and A. Drewnowski. 2004. "Clarifying Concepts about Macronutrients' Effects on Satiation and Satiety." *Journal of the American Dietetic Association* 104 (7):1151–53.

Harding, A.-H., L. A. Sargeant, A. Welch, S. Oakes, R. N. Luben, S. Bingham, N. E. Day, K.-T. Khaw, and N. J. Wareham. 2001. "Fat Consumption and HbA1c Levels: The EPIC-Norfolk Study." *Diabetes Care* 24 (11):1911–16.

Jenkins, D. J., C. W. Kendall, A. R. Josse, S. Salvatore, F. Brighenti, L. S. Augustin, P. R. Ellis, E. Vidgen, and A. V. Rao. 2006. "Almonds Decrease Postprandial Glycemia, Insulinemia, and Oxidative Damage in Healthy Individuals." *Journal of Nutrition* 136 (12):2987–92.

Jiang, R., J. E. Manson, M. J. Stampfer, S. Liu, W. C. Willett, and F. B. Hu. 2002. "Nut and Peanut Butter Consumption and Risk of Type 2 Diabetes in Women." *Journal of the American Medical Association* 288 (20):2554–60.

Kiyici, S., C. Ersoy, O. Oz Gul, E. Sarandol, M. Demirci, E. Tuncel, D. Sigirli, E. Erturk, and S. Imamoglu. 2009. "Total and Acylated Ghrelin Levels in Type 2 Diabetic Patients: Similar Levels Observed after Treatment with Metformin, Pioglitazone, or Diet Therapy." *Experimental and Clinical Endocrinology and Diabetes* 117 (8):386–90.

Kris-Etherton, P. M., W. S. Harris, and L. J. Appel. 2002. "Fish Consumption, Fish Oil, Omega-3 Fatty Acids, and Cardiovascular Disease." *Circulation* 106:2747–57.

Kusaka, I., S. Nagasaka, H. Horie, and S. Ishibashi. 2008. "Metformin, but Not Pioglitazone, Decreases Postchallenge Plasma Ghrelin Levels in Type 2 Diabetic Patients: A Possible Role in Weight Stability?" *Diabetes, Obesity, and Metabolism* 10 (11):1039–46.

Lemmer, J. T., D. E. Hurlbut, G. F. Martel, B. L. Tracy, F. M. Ivey, E. J. Metter, J. L. Fozard, J. L. Fleg, and B. F. Hurley. 2000. "Age and Gender Responses to Strength Training and Detraining." *Medicine and Science in Sports and Exercise* 32 (8):1505–12.

Lichtenstein, A. H., L. J. Appel, M. Brands, M. Carnethon, S. Daniels, H. A. Franch, B. Franklin, P. Kris-Etherton, W. S. Harris, B. Howard, N. Karanja, M. Lefevre, L. Rudel, F. Sacks, L. van Horn, M. Winston, and J. Wylie-Rosett. 2006. "Diet and Lifestyle Recommendations Revision 2006: A Scientific Statement from the American Heart Association Nutrition Committee." *Circulation* 114:82–96.

The Look AHEAD Research Group. 2010. "Long-term Effects of a Lifestyle Intervention on Weight and Cardiovascular Risk Factors in Individuals with Type 2 Diabetes Mellitus, Four-Year Results of the Look AHEAD Trial." Archives Internal Medicine 170 (17):1566-1575.American Heart Association Nutrition Committee." *Circulation* 114:82–96.

Maddalozzo, G. F., J. J. Widrick, B. J. Cardinal, K. M. Winters-Stone, M. A. Hoffman, and C. M. Snow. 2007. "The Effects of Hormone Replacement Therapy and Resistance Training on Spine Bone Mineral Density in Early Postmenopausal Women." *Bone* 40 (5):1244–51.

National Diabetes Information Clearinghouse (NDIC). 2008. "Diabetes Prevention Program." NIH Publication no. 09-5099. Bethesda, MD: U.S. Department of Health and Human Services National Institute of Diabetes and Digestive and Kidney Diseases, and National Institutes of Health. diabetes.niddk.nih.gov/dm/pubs/preventionprogram/ (accessed September 13, 2011).

———. 2011. "National Diabetes Statistics, 2011: Fast Facts on Diabetes." NIH Publication no. 11-3892. Bethesda, MD: U.S. Department of Health and Human Services National Institute of Diabetes and Digestive and Kidney Diseases, and National Institutes of Health.

Oldham-Cooper, R. E., C. A. Hardman, C. E. Nicoll, P. J. Rogers, and J. M. Brunstrom. 2011. "Playing a Computer Game during Lunch Affects Fullness, Memory for Lunch, and Later Snack Intake." *American Journal of Clinical Nutrition* 93 (2):308–13.

Pignone, M., M. J. Alberts, J. A. Colwell, M. Cushman, S. E. Inzucchi, D. Mukherjee, R. S. Rosenson, C. D. Williams, P. W. Wilson, and M. S. Kirkman. 2010. "Aspirin for Primary Prevention of Cardiovascular Events in People with Diabetes: A Position Statement of the American Diabetes Association, a Scientific Statement of the American Heart Association, and an Expert Consensus Document of the American College of Cardiology Foundation." *Circulation* 121 (24):2694–701.

Pinelli, N. R., A. Jantz, Z. Smith, A. Abouhassan, Christina Ayar, N. A. Jaber, A. W. Clarke, R. L. Commissaris, and L. A. Jaber. 2011. "Effect of Administration Time of Exenatide on Satiety Responses, Blood Glucose, and Adverse Events in Healthy Volunteers." *Journal of Clinical Pharmacology* 51 (2):165–72.

Sigal, R. J., G. P. Kenny, D. H. Wasserman, and C. Castaneda-Sceppa. 2004. "Physical Activity/Exercise and Type 2 Diabetes." *Diabetes Care* 27 (10):2518–39.

Sigal, R. J., G. P. Kenny, D. H. Wasserman, C. Castaneda-Sceppa, and R. D. White. 2006. "Physical Activity/Exercise and Type 2 Diabetes: A Consensus Statement from the American Diabetes Association." *Diabetes Care* 29 (6):1433–38. doi:10.2337/dc06-9910.

United States Department of Agriculture (USDA). 2010. *Dietary Guidelines for Americans, 2010*. www.dietaryguidelines.gov.

Wheeler, M. L., X. Pi-Sunyer. 2008. "Carbohydrate Issues: Type and Amount." *Journal American Dietetic Association* (ADA). 2008; 108:S34-S39.

Wien, M., D. Bleich, M. Raghuwanshi, S. Gould-Forgerite, J. Gomes, L. Monahan-Couch, and K. Oda. 2010. "Almond Consumption and Cardiovascular Risk Factors in Adults with Prediabetes." *Journal of the American College of Nutrition* 29 (3):189–97.

Wolf, G., and E. Ritz. 2005. "Combination Therapy with ACE Inhibitors and Angiotensin II Receptor Blockers to Halt Progression of Chronic Renal Disease: Pathophysiology and Indications." *Kidney International* 67 (3):799–812.

Index

I

JKL

M

XYZ

Michelle May, MD, is a recovered yo-yo dieter and founder of Am I Hungry?® Mindful Eating Workshops and Facilitator Training Program. She empowers individuals to end mindless and emotional eating without deprivation or guilt. An inspirational speaker and author, her passion and insight stem from her own personal struggles and her professional experiences helping thousands of people eat what they love and love what they eat. She lives in Phoenix, AZ.

Megrette Fletcher, MEd, RD, CDE, is a registered dietitian, certified diabetes educator, and internationally recognized mindful eating expert living north of Boston, MA. She is a cofounder of The Center for Mindful Eating. www.tcme.org

MORE BOOKS *from*
NEW HARBINGER PUBLICATIONS

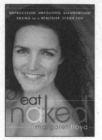

EAT NAKED
Unprocessed, Unpolluted &
Undressed Eating for a
Healthier, Sexier You

US $16.95 / ISBN: 978-1608820139
*Also available as an e-book
at newharbinger.com*

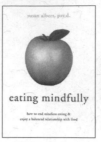

EATING MINDFULLY
How to End Mindless Eating
& Enjoy a Balanced
Relationship with Food

US $15.95 / ISBN: 978-1572243507
*Also available as an e-book
at newharbinger.com*

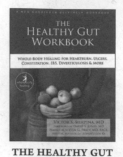

THE HEALTHY GUT
WORKBOOK
Whole-Body Healing for
Heartburn, Ulcers, Constipation,
IBS, Diverticulosis & More

US $21.95 / ISBN: 978-1572248441
*Also available as an e-book
at newharbinger.com*

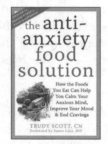

THE ANTIANXIETY
FOOD SOLUTION
How the Foods You Eat Can
Help You Calm Your Anxious
Mind, Improve Your Mood
& End Cravings

US $17.95 / ISBN: 978-1572249257
*Also available as an e-book
at newharbinger.com*

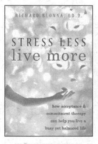

STRESS LESS,
LIVE MORE
How Acceptance &
Commitment Therapy Can
Help You Live a Busy yet
Balanced Life

US $16.95 / ISBN: 978-1572247093
*Also available as an e-book
at newharbinger.com*

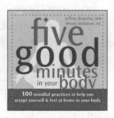

FIVE GOOD MINUTES®
IN YOUR BODY
100 Mindful Practices to Help
You Accept Yourself & Feel
at Home in Your Body

US $15.95 / ISBN: 978-1572245969
*Also available as an e-book
at newharbinger.com*

newharbingerpublications, inc.
1-800-748-6273 / newharbinger.com

 Like us on Facebook

 Follow us on Twitter
@newharbinger.com

(VISA, MC, AMEX / prices subject to change without notice)

Don't miss out on new books in the subjects that interest you.
Sign up for our **Book Alerts** at **newharbinger.com**

Check out www.psychsolve.com

Psych*Solve*® offers help with diagnosis, including treatment information on mental health
issues, such as depression, bipolar disorder, anxiety, phobias, stress and trauma,
relationship problems, eating disorders, chronic pain, and many other disorders.